CHRONIC PAIN
and OPIOID
MANAGEMENT

CHRONIC PAIN and OPIOID MANAGEMENT

Strategies for Integrated Treatment

Jennifer L. Murphy
Samantha Rafie

AMERICAN PSYCHOLOGICAL ASSOCIATION

Published by
American Psychological Association
750 First Street, NE
Washington, DC 20002
https://www.apa.org

Order Department
https://www.apa.org/pubs/books
order@apa.org

In the U.K., Europe, Africa, and the Middle East, copies may be ordered from Eurospan
https://www.eurospanbookstore.com/apa
info@eurospangroup.com

Typeset in Charter and Interstate by Circle Graphics, Inc., Reisterstown, MD

Printer: Sheridan Books, Chelsea, MI
Cover Designer: Publishers' Design and Production Services, Inc., Sagamore Beach, MA

Library of Congress Cataloging-in-Publication Data

Names: Murphy, Jennifer L., author. | Rafie, Samantha, author. |
  American Psychological Association, issuing body.
Title: Chronic pain and opioid management : strategies for integrated treatment /
  Jennifer L. Murphy and Samantha Rafie.
Description: Washington : American Psychological Association, [2020] |
  Includes bibliographical references and index.
Identifiers: LCCN 2020012228 (print) | LCCN 2020012229 (ebook) |
  ISBN 9781433832567 (paperback) | ISBN 9781433833946 (ebook)
Subjects: LCSH: Chronic pain—Treatment. | Opioids—Therapeutic use.
Classification: LCC RB127.5.C48 M87 2020 (print) | LCC RB127.5.C48 (ebook) |
  DDC 616/.0472—dc23
LC record available at https://lccn.loc.gov/2020012228
LC ebook record available at https://lccn.loc.gov/2020012229

https://doi.org/10.1037/0000209-000

Printed in the United States of America

10 9 8 7 6 5 4 3 2 1

To our patients, past, present, and future, who live bravely with chronic pain every day.

For Don and Jack—You are my reason.
—Jen

To my love and my sis, thank you for inspiring me to be and do my best.
—Sam

Contents

Foreword

In *Chronic Pain and Opioid Management: Strategies for Integrated Treatment*, Dr. Jennifer L. Murphy and Dr. Samantha Rafie, both nationally well-regarded and experienced clinical and research pain psychologists, teach health care providers how to give effective, comprehensive care to patients struggling with chronic pain who are also on prescribed opioids. This manual is not about how to taper or deprescribe but rather is a patient-centric guide for how to collaboratively prepare patients for positive behavioral change, engage patients in change strategies, and help patients maintain the gains they have made, however incrementally small those gains are.

This is a must-read text for not only practicing clinical psychologists but also for all of us with clinical practices who encounter patients struggling with persistent pain. I know this well, having been a primary care general internal medicine physician since 1982 and a board-certified pain specialist since 1995. In my current position, I have had the unique opportunity to interact with literally thousands of primary care clinicians: physicians, nurses, advanced practice providers, pharmacists, social workers, and health psychologists who care for complex patients with chronic pain, many of whom have been on opioids for decades. I've heard firsthand of the challenges to pain care delivery from hundreds of frontline practice sites via traditional in-person consultations. And having just read this book, I can confidently state that Dr. Murphy and Dr. Rafie have made an important contribution to the field of pain medicine, a contribution that enables us to do better for all of our patients who struggle with chronic pain, and in particular those on long-term opioids.

A bit of history will help to contextualize the book's contribution to the field. Over the past several decades, two paradigm shifts have deeply affected the science and management of pain. Our first modern understanding of pain was formulated in 1953 by John Bonica in his comprehensive textbook, *The Management of Pain* (Bonica, 1990). Dr. Bonica, an anesthesiologist, and his colleague Dr. Wilbur Fordyce, a clinical psychologist, emphasized the importance of our patients' psychological and social experiences and established the biopsychosocial model necessary for understanding and treating pain, a still undisputed foundational principle of pain management. The earliest best practice for assessing and treating pain required understanding our individual patients' psychological states and social environments. This was and is considered multidisciplinary pain management. It briefly flourished.

The first paradigm shift occurred in the 1990s. Chronic pain treatment became more and more reliant on a purely biomedical approach, which included a heavy use of drugs, devices, and procedural interventions. Among the many causes for this move away from pain's psychological and social determinants was a complex mix of strictly nonmedical factors, including but not limited to the shifting economics of health care delivery (which leave inadequate time to provide needed care), the pharmaceutical industry's substantial development and promotion of new oral opioids, and insufficient pain education and training for students and postlicensure professionals in medical and other health sciences.

At the time, opioids were even less well understood than they are today. Gaps remain in our knowledge of mechanisms of tolerance and craving; opioid receptor actions and biases; limits to opioid and other drug efficacy; hyperalgesia and central sensitization; and the neurobiology and co-occurrence of opioid misuse, behavioral health disorders, and substance use disorders. As a famous quote attributed to Voltaire says, "Physicians pour drugs of which they know little, for diseases of which they know less, into patients of which they know nothing at all." Although today's doctors know much more about health and medicine than did doctors in the mid-18th century (when Voltaire lived), we are still far from mastering our art and science.

In this shift from a biopsychosocial approach to a primarily biomedical approach, opioid use expanded beyond acute perioperative care, palliative end-of-life care, and cancer pain. Many patients and their prescribers believed that opioids were their best or even only option for pain management; indeed, I readily recall many of my own patients asking, "Do I have to be dying of cancer to get pain care?" New extended-release opioids were becoming commercially available, and doctors increasingly prescribed them because it took less time and energy to write a prescription than to listen to patients; to educate them about the nature of chronic pain, the risks of long-term opioid use, and the value of using behavioral health care to manage pain; and to navigate these patients to appropriate behavioral health care. Furthermore, during this period, most insurance coverage for nonbiomedical care went from little to nothing at all. The biomedical approach promised quick fixes to pain, and it was thus supported by all parties: patients, doctors, third-party payers, industry, media, and a wide range of thought leaders and policymakers.

The biomedical approach overlooked the fundamental role of behavioral sciences in the management of pain. Why spend time and waste money on inconvenient and often unavailable, albeit well proven, pain treatment strategies such as cognitive behavioral therapy? Why even bother with the other less well studied yet still demonstrated-effective treatments, such as physical therapy? Patients don't want us to tell them that their "pain is all in their head." Who likes to go to physical therapy anyway, especially when a pill, or many pills, or an injection, or even surgery will cure their pain? And so-called nonscientific treatments—such as mindfulness-based stress reduction, yoga, tai chi, and acupuncture—were dismissed as luxury activities for people without "real pain."

But another paradigm shift is occurring now, and it is a response to the health crisis that resulted from the last paradigm. That health crisis is the opioid epidemic, a combination of drug abuse and overprescribing that has claimed far more American lives in 2 years than the entire Vietnam War (National Center for Health Statistics, 2020). Annual deaths from opioid overdose now exceed those at the peak of the AIDS epidemic (GBD 2015 HIV Collaborators, 2016). Over the past 3 years, life expectancy in the United States has dropped for the first time ever recorded (Woolf & Schoomaker, 2019), largely as a result of the "diseases of despair," led by opioid overdoses, alcoholism, and death by suicide. Over 200,000 people have died from overdoses that involve opioids, and until recently, predominantly clinician-prescribed opioids led these poisonings. Guidelines, such as from the Centers for Disease Control and Prevention (CDC; Dowell et al., 2016), and widely embraced state laws and disciplinary rules have begun to affect opioid prescribing practices dramatically. Many patients who have been on prescribed opioids for decades—many of whom are on high doses and often in combination with potent sedatives—are left hopeless, seeing few if any alternatives. As a result, the health care field is beginning to shift back to the earlier paradigm of biopsychosocial care. There is renewed interest in learning how best to reimagine and redeploy behavioral therapies and how best to provide an enriched approach to the advancing methods that improve the psychosocial health of our patients with pain. As I've known since John Bonica and Wilbur Fordyce taught me in 1980, pain treated comprehensively requires a biopsychosocial approach.

Guidelines now insist that the initial treatment of pain is with nondrug options. CDC Guideline #1 begins, "Nonpharmacologic therapy and nonopioid pharmacologic therapy are preferred for chronic pain" (Dowell et al., 2016). There is now explicit emphasis on self-management strategies. Here in Washington State, new 2019 opioid prescribing rules assert that

> the physician shall exercise their professional judgment in selecting appropriate treatment modalities for acute nonoperative, acute perioperative, subacute, or chronic pain including the use of multimodal pharmacologic and *nonpharmacologic therapy* [emphasis added] as an alternative to opioids whenever reasonable, clinically appropriate, evidence-based alternatives exist. (Washington Administrative Code, 2019)

We are now not only advised but legally required to treat pain "comprehensively." Patient self-management is increasingly valued, and clinicians are prompted to engage in shared decision making. This type of care mandates a biopsychosocial approach. Law- and rule-making authorities now require that doctors consider cognitive behavioral therapy and sleep hygiene for treating chronic pain.

So here is where Murphy and Rafie's *Chronic Pain and Opioid Management: Strategies for Integrated Treatment* becomes an essential text. In this book, the authors present evidence-based psychological treatments supported by the most up-to-date research, including motivational interviewing, cognitive and behavioral therapy, acceptance and commitment therapy, and mindfulness-based stress reduction. The authors cover an array of important topics, including the stigma, anger, frustration, and hopelessness and helplessness of our patients. They emphasize active listening, empathy, support, and patient education. As they state, "With proper education, the foundation for self-management of chronic pain is set." The authors also address the prescriber's own guilt and sense of responsibility to help ease the suffering of others. Chapter 6 is especially useful for the many primary care clinicians who do not have access to trained clinical psychologists because it provides step-by-step instructions for developing an integrated treatment plan, focusing on activity pacing and goal setting. Throughout the book, strategies are illustrated by brief, realistic example scenarios labeled Clinical Conundrums. Problem solving, goal setting, and interview techniques are all covered. At the end of the book is a list of additional resources.

For these reasons, I wholeheartedly recommend this exceptionally worth-while book to read, absorb, and implement into practice for physicians, behavioral health providers, and all other members of the pain management treatment team. I'll conclude with some salient words of Maya Angelou (1994): "Do the best you can until you know better. Then when you know better, do better." Now is the time for us to get knowing.

—*David J. Tauben, MD, FACP*
University of Washington, Seattle

Preface

We had the good fortune of starting our careers by training and working in the inpatient Chronic Pain Rehabilitation Program at the Tampa VA. Although we did not fully realize or appreciate it at the time, this treatment setting represents the ideal version of biopsychosocially driven, team-based chronic pain care. Program participants are tapered off of opioids in a structured, safe, and supportive environment while exploring all of the factors that impact their pain experience. Over the course of the program, they are equipped with active strategies to take control of their pain and their lives. In this context, it was normal and expected to incorporate behavioral strategies for pain and opioid management into integrated interventions, as had been done for decades.

As the opioid crisis unfolded, starting in the late 1990s and increasing enormously in the 2010s, behavioral management during tapering became a topic of keen interest, and resources to help guide these often challenging clinical situations were limited. During this period, our presentations on the topic of behavioral considerations for opioid tapering were frequently followed by clinicians inquiring about additional resources, research, and sources of information. Unfortunately, there was little to share. Similar issues have arisen when we train clinicians in the use of cognitive behavioral therapy for chronic pain. Health care practitioners routinely share an urgently felt need to implement behavioral approaches for pain, given opioid-related concerns and deprescribing realities in their practice settings. They want to provide a collaborative and therapeutic environment where both chronic pain and opioid concerns can be addressed. This desire extends beyond mental or behavioral health clinicians—the need is felt across the continuum of care, from prescribers to physical therapists, nurses to chiropractors. Most helping professionals have been touched directly by the public health crises of chronic pain and opioids and want to do something to make it better.

Through this book, we wanted to acknowledge the reality of the challenging issues that patients and providers face every day and to offer guidance for how to optimize outcomes during these often complex clinical interactions. Our broad-based professional efforts—including direct patient care, funded research trials, and system-wide leadership—have focused on how to leverage evidence-based behavioral pain medicine interventions to improve pain management and decrease the use of treatment options with higher risk. We have seen the life-changing effects that can occur when individuals with pain are listened to, believed in, and partnered with. Even for the most downtrodden, transformation is always possible. The strategies shared here can be used to assure individuals who may feel at the mercy of pain and opioids that they are not alone; there are treatments that can help. We hope that this book provides strong practices that are beneficial to other health care providers and that these approaches will enable your patients to live their best lives.

While we have no way to thank all the patients who have shared their stories, time, and energy, we are humbled by the privilege of being let into your lives. We would like to acknowledge the esteemed leaders in behavioral pain medicine and interdisciplinary pain care, who have been providing clinical models and informative research on what good pain care looks like for many decades; these leaders continue to push for behavioral treatment to be incorporated into guidelines and practice, and there is much work to be done. Our appreciation goes to the American Psychological Association for supporting this book and to our editor, Beth Hatch, for her patience and insights with polishing. Thank you to Michael H. Craine, PhD, for his thoughtful comments on the book, as well as to the other expert reviewers who shared valuable suggestions for refinement and revision.

Jennifer L. Murphy would like to extend her deepest gratitude to Michael E. Clark, PhD, for providing mentorship and the opportunity to learn how to help people with chronic pain before she knew it was her calling. He demonstrated that you must stand for something or you will fall for anything, a sentiment that resonates almost daily in this work. She would like to thank the many talented multidisciplinary health care professionals with whom she has had the great benefit of working with and growing from in clinical, research, and leadership roles. Jennifer would also like to acknowledge the steadfast support and love of her family throughout her educational and professional endeavors, including this book. Finally, she would like to thank her coauthor for being the perfect partner in this journey and for pushing her to finish when a nudge would not have done.

Samantha Rafie would like to recognize the wisdom imparted by colleagues, supervisors, and mentors from current and past teams across the United States, all of whom had such an immense impact on her development, both professionally and personally. Samantha would like to express great appreciation for the encouragement and patience of her family during the book writing process and beyond and for being the team behind the scenes through the many phases of this path. Finally, Samantha would like to thank her coauthor, colleague, and friend for years of support and for carving the way for others.

CHRONIC PAIN
and OPIOID
MANAGEMENT

INTRODUCTION

To address the opioid crisis in the United States, leaders in pain care and public health have joined in a widespread effort to curtail the less-than-judicious prescribing of opioid analgesics. Updated clinical practice guidelines increased regulation of prescriptions, and educational outreach helped to decrease serious adverse events related to prescription opioids, including overdose deaths. This effort is an undeniable positive (Johnson et al., 2018). Unfortunately, opioid-related concerns have also been the impetus for a focus on drug management instead of pain management, and people with pain have often suffered because their doctors focused solely on reducing or eliminating opioids. Emphasizing safety in prescribing is critical; however, offering individualized and compassionate care for those who are suffering is also built into the duty to do no harm.

Although most patients using opioids for chronic pain have not misused them, many have developed an overreliance on these medications because opioid properties lead to physical dependence and tolerance. In recent years, too often patients have had their medications changed with limited explanation regarding dose adjustments and have had few options to manage

https://doi.org/10.1037/0000209-001
Chronic Pain and Opioid Management: Strategies for Integrated Treatment,
by J. L. Murphy and S. Rafie

suffering. The authors of the Centers for Disease Control and Prevention guideline for prescribing opioids for chronic pain (Dowell et al., 2016) have acknowledged that the guidelines have been misapplied and used in ways beyond their original intent (Dowell et al., 2019). Thus, those with pain are caught in the middle of a societal and political maelstrom in which the headlining opioid epidemic has blurred the line between those who have been prescribed opioids for pain management and those who use opioids illegally (e.g., using heroin or fentanyl; National Academies of Sciences, Engineering, & Medicine, 2017). Signs from suffering protestors read, "Don't punish pain." Unexpected changes in opioid medication may indeed feel like punishment to individuals who have received minimal education about the limitations of pharmaceuticals in chronic pain management and do not fully understand what is needed to achieve optimal functioning as well as analgesia.

The experiences of patients and providers at the intersection of chronic pain and opioids demand more strategies and research for improved management of both concerns. An upside to the stream of negative opioid-related events is increased interest in nonpharmacological approaches to chronic pain management. *Relieving Pain in America: A Blueprint for Transforming Prevention, Care, Education, and Research* (Institute of Medicine, 2011) called for a "cultural transformation" (p. 2) for pain care in the United States. This report led to major developments in 2016, when both the *National Pain Strategy* (U.S. Office of the Assistant Secretary for Health, 2016) and the *CDC Guideline for Prescribing Opioids for Chronic Pain* (Dowell et al., 2016) were released. Taken together, these publications provide a firm statement that chronic pain is a biopsychosocial condition and must be "treated with integrated, multimodal, interdisciplinary, evidence-based approaches" (U.S. Office of the Assistant Secretary for Health, 2016, p. 3), and that "nonpharmacologic therapy and nonopioid pharmacologic therapy are preferred. . . . If opioids are used, they should be combined with non-pharmacologic therapy and nonopioid pharmacologic therapy, as appropriate" (Dowell et al., 2016). Additional guidelines indicate that optimal treatment should incorporate a variety of options from movement to mindfulness to address pain adequately (Dowell et al., 2016; U.S. Department of Veterans Affairs and Department of Defense, 2017).

Behavioral treatments for chronic pain are not new, and some, such as cognitive behavioral therapy, are backed by decades of research supporting their effectiveness (Eccleston et al., 2013; Ehde et al., 2014; Morley et al., 1999; Skelly et al., 2018). Despite this, the term "pain management" is often synonymous with pharmacology and biomedical approaches only, driven in part by the never-ending quest for a simple medical fix. This tendency ignores the reality that chronic pain is a complex condition requiring a comprehensive approach and has no magic bullet. One of the primary problems is that pain is generally understood in terms of an acute or short-term issue; however, chronic pain is a very different phenomenon. Chronic pain cannot be solved with an opioid or any single treatment modality. It is an ongoing condition that must be managed over time, much like Type 2 diabetes—both medical intervention and various behavioral choices affect the trajectory of the disease and its resulting impacts.

Chronic pain conditions are multifactorial and complex on their own; once opioid use is part of the clinical picture, the layers of biopsychosocial considerations grow exponentially. The resulting situation can be challenging for providers to address adequately, as such individuals typically require a higher level of care and treatments that address multiple concerns. Unfortunately, little empirical data are currently available on integrated interventions for pain and opioid use issues. While there is sufficient evidence to create a clear map for addressing the psychosocial factors of pain, there is a gap in the literature on best practices and a shortage of clinical resources for those with a more complex constellation of symptoms. Better pain treatments are important for curtailing the opioid concerns, but if we try to address only pain without considering the role of opioids in patients' experiences, we are not being honest or complete in our approach.

Typically, treatment settings are aimed at either pain or opioids, but not both, and it is not uncommon to be denied pain treatment options in the presence of opioid concerns. Too often, fingers are pointed from one treatment area to another—providers whose focus is addressing opioid misuse convey the message "If you could get the patient's pain under control, then we wouldn't have these problems!" Similarly, pain specialists refer patients who use opioids to a substance abuse clinic, seeking to disown the complications of problems such as opioid use disorder (OUD) even though pain remains a pressing concern for the person who attended the appointment hoping for relief. In addition, those in settings such as primary care or community-based clinics regularly encounter patients who are struggling with both pain and opioid issues. These practitioners may feel particularly underprepared to provide useful interventions given their usual lack of time and their focus on generalist training. And sadly, research indicates that those with substance use disorders are less likely than others to receive effective pain treatment (Rupp & Delaney, 2004).

WHY THIS BOOK?

The purpose of this book is to offer health care providers a contextual framework and implementable, integrated strategies to assist those individuals managing both chronic pain and opioids. In the literature, these issues are often addressed separately; however, that separation does not reflect the realities of clinical practice. It is now commonplace to encounter patients who have longstanding chronic pain and are in the process of addressing their opioid use. Some may be tapering opioids slowly with few negative effects and may be pleased with the decrease in medication use. Others may have been urged by a prescriber to reduce their opioids and may feel highly resistant to the idea, even in the absence of significant analgesic or functional benefit. Still others may be self-motivated to decrease opioids but fearful about how such a change might impact their pain or their lives.

The situation is complicated for both patient and health care provider and is often accompanied by a multifaceted clinical picture that includes medical and psychiatric comorbidities as the backdrop. Given that, it is both efficient and sensible to integrate discussions and guidance regarding how all the relevant pieces fit together. Conjointly discussing pain and opioid management from an integrated behavioral standpoint is useful as it embraces a whole-person approach to care, allows cross-cutting strategies to be applied, and maximizes the reduction of suffering. One of the limitations of currently supported behavioral treatment options is that they do not explicitly incorporate considerations related to the use of opioids. For many who need assistance, particularly those with high-impact pain, these issues are inextricably linked and should be treated as such, hence the effort to do just that.

This is a book on better treatment for those individuals with chronic pain who are at one of the many points along the opioid journey: considering deprescribing, in the process of opioid tapering, having recently discontinued opioids, or using opioids effectively for pain, among others. They are suffering from the effects of chronic pain, and opioids have been an important or at least a familiar part of life. We (the authors) are experts in pain management and have seen firsthand the utility of integrating effective clinical communication and behavioral strategies related to these issues. We are not addictionologists or addiction therapists, but we have been exposed to far more challenges regarding opioid use, misuse, addiction, and dependence than anticipated because we came of age in the current health care landscape. Learning to weave together the clinical approaches for both pain and opioid concerns is part of the art of optimizing treatment.

This book is not aimed specifically at opioid tapering. Whether or not to taper opioids is a decision that is made ultimately between the prescribing medical provider and the person with pain. With the patient's consent, loved ones should be involved in the process because they are affected by the decision, can be helped by education and expectations around deprescribing, and are instrumental in whether decreasing is successful or not. Health care providers, such as nurses, psychologists, and other members of the pain treatment team, can provide information and support for individuals tapering at every stage, integrated pain and opioid strategies for optimizing these interactions are thus useful to all parties. If indicated, reductions in opioid use should be planned thoughtfully and in a collaborative manner. Unless there is an urgent safety need, it is appropriate for an individual to taper opioids slowly on an outpatient basis, check in regularly, and monitor effects on functioning.

This book is also not about OUD. It is critically important to evaluate every person who uses opioids and determine if they have OUD. While most will not, those who do or likely do must be connected with a clinical pathway where they can access appropriate, evidence-based options for OUD such as medication-assisted treatment (MAT). Ideally, access to MAT is without significant barriers, and there is an established process to facilitate a "warm handoff." Once a mechanism for addressing opioid dependence is implemented, ways to behaviorally manage chronic pain and familiar desires for opioids are likely to emerge. The strategies outlined here would likely be helpful for these individuals as well, in conjunction with other indicated treatments for substance use such as addiction-focused counseling.

Patients who are balancing pain and opioid use are prevalent across the spectrum of health care services and are treated by individuals from various disciplines in a range of settings. The approaches in this book, therefore, are intended to assist any practitioner who can be helped by better understanding the population, improving rapport and engagement, and implementing useful treatment strategies. It has been said many times that pain is a team sport—it is best managed not by physicians alone but by a group of multidisciplinary providers. To provide the best care, this book can be used by a range of those individuals, including but not limited to

- *behavioral health clinicians* (e.g., psychologists, social workers, counselors): Those in behavioral health must take a leadership role in addressing how all aspects of patients' lives impact and are impacted by chronic pain and opioid use. They can help empower patients by providing tools for increased self-efficacy.

- *physicians and prescribing medical providers* (e.g., MD, DO, advance practice nurse, PA): Pain is the most common presenting complaint for medical providers working in primary care settings and for many specialists. Their communication and input regarding the best approaches for pain and opioids is foundational and often holds much weight with patients.

- *nurses*: Nurses are often the front line to health care. Seen in primary and specialty care, they are gatekeepers to all things related to the patient's health. Their importance cannot be overestimated; it is, therefore, particularly critical for them to have the knowledge and skills to best assist this population.

- *physical medicine and rehabilitation therapists*: Physical, occupational, vocational, and recreational therapists as well as others interface routinely with this patient population and may feel underprepared. Their functional restoration focus leaves them well positioned to enhance their clinical effectiveness by adding helpful approaches.

- *pharmacists*: Clinical pharmacists are increasingly involved in pain management generally and in plans for prescribing opioids more specifically. They increasingly offer consultative assistance to providers and interact with patients in settings that range from the community pharmacy to the multidisciplinary hospital team.

- *complementary and integrative health care professionals*: Options such as chiropractic care, yoga, tai chi, acupuncture, and massage are increasingly in demand for this population. Practitioners can bolster their approaches by incorporating integrated pain and opioid strategies in a setting where patients are often comfortable and open.

OVERVIEW OF THIS BOOK

This book is divided into four parts. Part I, Foundations (Chapters 1–3), provides an overview of terminology and definitions, theoretical underpinnings, and empirical background necessary to understand the rationale and presentation of the approaches for pain and opioid management that follow. Many of the hesitations and fears that individuals possess can be assuaged with outcomes from others in similar positions; therefore, it is helpful for providers to be acquainted with the data. The Foundations section also explores the relationship between patient and provider, which is critical across health care conditions but deserves special attention among a clinical population that often feels misunderstood.

Following this important background information, the focus of the book shifts to clinical guidance, and the remaining three parts describe three phases of treatment. Although treatment is presented in a linear fashion, the reality of clinical care is that most patients move in a more fluid manner between topics or stages. Motivation, pain, stressors, and setbacks wax and wane, so health care providers should anticipate the need for ongoing assessment and flexibility over time.

Part II, Phase 1: Preparing for Change (Chapters 4 and 5), focuses on readying the patient for treatment. Particularly for those managing the difficulties that arise with chronic pain and opioid use, a proper evaluation to identify the presence of OUD is critical. Exploring past experiences and potential resistances to behavioral treatment and possible changes in opioid regimen must be handled with openness and directness.

Part III, Phase 2: Engaging in Strategies (Chapters 6–9), is about involving the patient in making behavioral changes by using the collaborative development of goals and a pathway for treatment. Specific integrated approaches are introduced, with clinical examples provided. These strategies will help with both pain and the anxieties that surface when one is managing opioids. This section also elucidates how to troubleshoot issues with implementation of skills and how to address potential symptoms that arise during treatment.

Part IV, Phase 3: Maintaining Gains (Chapters 10–12), focuses on maintenance of gains. While many patients are able to make changes, sustaining change over the long term can be the greatest challenge. This section of the book includes information about how to develop a concrete plan to guide behavior, establish realistic expectations for the future, and optimize resources to stay on track and minimize setbacks.

For all three phases, we illustrate concepts using a fictional patient named Jim. In sections labeled "Clinical Conundrum," we describe Jim's challenges and strengths and present a dialogue between Jim and his health care provider. Jim is first introduced in Chapter 4, and he reappears in subsequent chapters to demonstrate common concerns and reactions from patients as well as sample responses for providers. As Jim progresses through treatment, readers are introduced to recommended techniques appropriate to the context and stage of change. These Clinical Conundrum sections are important learning tools as providers consider how to use an approach with real patients.

LANGUAGE CHOICES

A note about terminology is in order. The words that we choose when discussing health conditions can be powerful and make an impact in positive or negative directions. This can be especially true when writing or speaking about topics that may be inherently sensitive, such as substance use. Stating that someone is an "opioid abuser," for example, sounds pejorative and blaming; however, a "person with an opioid use disorder" shifts the focus to the behavior and away from the individual, and this shift can be helpful (Kelly et al., 2010). Furthermore, a term such as "opioid misuse" may have a better connotation when interacting with patients and may lead to improved communication. When characterized as a "drug seeker" during a visit to the doctor, many patients feel they have been reduced to a stereotype, not listened to as a human being who is in great discomfort. Although far less often acknowledged, this situation also frequently occurs with individuals experiencing chronic pain. Describing someone in the health care system as a "pain patient" often implies unfavorable qualities about the individual—that they may be challenging to interact with or difficult to please. Providers may form prejudgments that set the stage for suboptimal clinical interactions. For this reason, we use the terms "people" and "individuals" when discussing those who are managing chronic pain and opioids. Their health conditions are not who they are but rather are one of many factors contributing to their whole self.

Along that line, perhaps the greatest challenge with this book was determining the best way to reference individuals' opioid use. Because this book is not intended exclusively for those who are tapering opioids but rather for a broader group at various stages with opioids, it was not possible to label the general population accurately with a simplistic term. Because our focus is not on those with OUD explicitly, we largely avoid this topic. And while we maintain the connection between chronic pain and opioids for consistent integration in treatment, we do not assume that everyone is misusing or taking medications other than as prescribed. Misuse may be an issue for some patients, but the focus of the book is an empathic, active, wellness-based approach to clinical interactions for a broad spectrum of clinical presentations.

I
FOUNDATIONS

INTRODUCTION

The pain experience is highly complex, and the understanding of it has evolved significantly in the last half century. Because pain is not solely physical or psychological but is a biopsychosocial phenomenon involving the whole person, health care providers must first appreciate the extensive factors that interact to constitute each individual's story. For many who seek relief from pain-related suffering, opioid analgesics are or have been a significant part of their narrative. While the details around pain can be challenging to convey to others, communication regarding opioid use can be even more difficult. To best serve those who are struggling, it is paramount to have the necessary background regarding factors affecting their experience.

This section provides the foundation that health care providers need for the treatment strategies used in this book. Although not presented as information that is to be used in a hands-on way, it provides the empirical background on which the rest of the book is built. Relevant definitions, theoretical underpinnings, and psychosocial factors are shared to create a context for the subsequent approaches. A literature review of psychobehavioral approaches known to be effective in chronic pain management as well as evidence regarding the process of opioid reduction is provided as a foundation for selected strategies. Finally, information about the critical patient–provider relationship is examined. The emphasis is on aspects that make clinical interactions more effective because establishing solid rapport is foundational in achieving optimal outcomes in pain and opioid management.

1 CHRONIC PAIN AND OPIOIDS

Before beginning a discussion about the clinical management of chronic pain and opioids, it is important to review basic definitions and theories that are relevant to understanding and applying the therapeutic content and approaches. This chapter provides foundational information regarding the evolution of pain conceptualization, which includes the recognition of psychosocial variables and their treatment as critical. The terminology and diagnostic domains surrounding opioids are also reviewed, with acknowledgment that some of the opioid-related topics are constantly changing and are often debated among health care providers. While a comprehensive review of chronic pain and opioids could be a book unto itself, this selective discussion is intended to highlight key topics that are important in creating a context for discussion of what may be unfamiliar behavioral strategies.

PAIN BASICS: A COMPLEX PHENOMENON

Pain is one of the most universal experiences, shared by all human beings and typically understood in terms of acute pain, which follows an injury,

https://doi.org/10.1037/0000209-002
Chronic Pain and Opioid Management: Strategies for Integrated Treatment,
by J. L. Murphy and S. Rafie

illness, surgery, or other identifiable event and resolves within approximately 3 months. While unpleasant, it is short term and there is an end in sight. For the most part, Americans' general understanding of pain reflects this linear pathway for pain treatment. When one seeks care from a health care provider for a pain complaint, the expectation is of learning first the "what"—what is this? Next is the "how"—how do we fix it, and how long will it take? And finally, the "thank you"—discomfort dissipates, patient is relieved, and provider is satisfied with the outcome. The experience and process of chronic pain are very different. *Chronic pain* lasts for longer than 3 months and continues beyond what might be expected in the cases of injury or illness. In chronic conditions such as degenerative disc disease or fibromyalgia, chronic pain is the rule from the beginning, as resolution is not expected.

Understandings of Pain

Theoretical frameworks regarding pain have shifted significantly over the centuries. In the 1600s, Rene Descartes (1972) hypothesized that pain was based on a mechanistic process connecting physiological processes. One of the first modern understandings of pain, and one of the most significant, was the specificity theory from Max von Frey in 1895 (as cited in Moayedi & Davis, 2013), who suggested a specific system of dedicated fibers that lead signals to a separate "pain center" in the brain. Research on touch receptors and a pain pathway in the spine appeared to lend credence to this idea (Rey, 1989), and the idea of pain as an independent sensation prevailed for over half a century. This understanding of pain supported the notion that a purely biomedical, unimodal approach could adequately address pain.

Psychological approaches for understanding and treating pain gained prominence in the 1960s with the revolutionary gate control theory of pain, introduced by Melzack and Wall (1965). Unlike the earlier understanding that pain was a simplistic and purely biological response, Melzack and Wall posited that psychosocial as well as physiological factors affect the processing of pain and therefore are built into the development and maintenance of chronic pain (cf. Melzack, 1999). Specifically, they stated that pain was a central nervous system phenomenon wherein sensory input from the periphery was modulated by motivational-affective and cognitive–evaluative influences. They also thoroughly discredited previous explanations of pain. Later, Melzack (2001) proposed the neuromatrix theory, arguing that the multidimensional experience of pain is informed by neurosignature patterns that may trigger sensory input but can also exist without them. This theory offered an additional useful framework to conceptualize the complex chronic pain experience.

More recent research builds on the foundations of Melzack and Wall (1965) and further supports the theory that pain is a complex experience requiring whole-person evaluation and treatment from multiple disciplines. A biopsychosocial model of pain emerged (Gatchel, 2005), which led to a still-growing body of empirical research related to understanding key behavioral, psychological, and social–contextual factors that influence the process of pain. The biopsychosocial model conceptualizes chronic pain as a condition that requires ongoing management strategies that consider the multifactorial experience (Gatchel, 2005). This model has been the single greatest support to a more comprehensive approach to adequately treat chronic pain, one that employs psychological interventions either as part of a larger, multidisciplinary pain management program or as a routine consult much like physical therapy.

Psychosocial Factors

Numerous psychosocial and behavioral variables are inextricably connected to the pain experience (Edwards, Dworkin, et al., 2016; Gatchel et al., 2007; Roditi & Robinson, 2011). Pain is by nature subjective, and although the way that people respond to pain is related to physiological factors, it is also influenced by a host of other factors, including cognitive appraisal, emotional state, and previous experience. One of the most disruptive factors in the pain experience is emotional distress; therefore, the role of negative emotions such as depression, anxiety, and general distress has been studied extensively in those with pain (Burke et al., 2015; Fernandez & Kerns, 2008). Estimates suggest that at least half of the people with chronic pain meet the criteria for depression (Bair et al., 2003), and the presence of depression in those with pain is associated with higher rates of disability and higher levels of pain intensity (Linton & Bergbom, 2011). Premorbid psychological dysfunction serves as a risk factor for the development of pain conditions (Fillingim, 2017). Furthermore, symptoms of emotional distress contribute strongly to pain treatment outcomes, even more strongly than pain intensity in many studies (Edwards, Dworkin, et al., 2016; Lerman et al., 2015). Individuals with chronic pain are at increased risk of suicide (Petrosky et al., 2018; Tang & Crane, 2006), with a third of those with chronic pain contemplating or attempting suicide at some point (Ilgen et al., 2008).

Traumatic experiences have also been widely studied, and strong prospective links have been observed between early traumas and pain

(Afari et al., 2014), as well as between combat exposure and posttraumatic stress disorder in adulthood (Asmundson & Katz, 2009; Brennstuhl et al., 2015). Not surprisingly, anxiety and worry are more common in those with pain, who also have higher rates of anxiety disorders (Asmundson & Katz, 2009). Pain catastrophizing, conceptualized as a negative cognitive–affective response to pain or anticipated pain (Quartana et al., 2009), has been shown to be one of the strongest psychological predictors of pain outcomes, with a substantial body of research indicating its key role in pain-related functioning and disability (Abbott et al., 2011; Thibault et al., 2008; Wertli, Eugster, et al., 2014; Wollaars et al., 2007). Its importance in pain processing and outcomes is significant and is explored in greater depth later in Chapter 2.

Behavioral Principles and Self-Regulatory Strategies

Much of behavioral treatment for those with pain remains rooted in Skinner's (1965) operant principles, which were applied to pain specifically by Fordyce (1976). These principles suggest that pain-related behaviors can be maintained or extinguished given reinforcement or a lack thereof. Behaviors can be "conditioned" over time if they are reinforced by desirable consequences. For example, various expressions of pain may lead loved ones to complete all household chores while insisting that the patient rest, providing both sympathy and support for avoidance of activity. Treatment might use similar operant principles by reinforcing behaviors that are more adaptive (e.g., graded activity engagement) to decrease those that are not beneficial (e.g., isolation). The fear-avoidance model (Vlaeyen & Linton, 2000) also relates to operant principles and is highly relevant to the chronic pain experience and treatment. It posits that when patients repeatedly believe that pain signals are dangerous, as is common in chronic conditions, they may engage in fear-driven avoidance behaviors and cognitions that lead to negative consequences (e.g., deconditioning, social withdrawal). Studies of thousands of people with low back pain (Wertli, Rasmussen-Barr, et al., 2014) suggest that high levels of fear-avoidance behaviors postinjury are associated with higher levels of pain and functional disability and poorer treatment outcomes overall. Depression is another factor influencing recovery postinjury, and it must be managed as part of the essential post-injury care (Kellezi et al., 2017). Treatments, therefore, are designed to decrease these errant beliefs by addressing behaviors and decreasing pain-related fears and cognitions, anxiety, and depression.

Over time, various approaches incorporating behavioral principles through a variety of lenses have emerged. The empirical data regarding the effectiveness of these behavioral treatments for pain are reviewed in Chapter 2.

The works of Melzack and Wall (1965) suggested that changing individuals' responses to pain would change their experience of pain. This research supported the notion that patients could take more control over pain management by acquiring skills to reduce its impact on them. Approaches that increase self-regulation link the processes of body and mind, acknowledging the whole-person connection. The focus is on increasing awareness of physiological states and better regulation of autonomic responses.

Various tools that are critical in the behavioral treatment of pain include relaxation techniques, biofeedback, and mindfulness. The details regarding these tools and their role in controlling pain will be explored in greater depth at various points throughout the book. Of note, recent studies have examined how cognitive self-regulation affects autonomic responses (Matthewson et al., 2019), suggesting that regulating cognitions affects both pain ratings and pain-related physiology. While relatively unexplored, this finding suggests another direction for future studies to support approaches that involve adaptations to pain-related cognitions.

OPIOIDS: DEFINITIONS AND KEY TERMS

An *opioid* is a natural or synthetic chemical that interacts with the opioid receptors on the nerve cells in the body and brain, reducing feelings of pain (U.S. Office of the Surgeon General, 2018). This class of drugs includes prescribed medications that are used for pain management, such as oxycodone and hydrocodone, as well as illicit drugs, such as heroin. Fentanyl, a synthetic opioid medication used for severe pain management, is considerably more potent than heroin and has been increasingly manufactured and sold illegally (Centers for Disease Control and Prevention [CDC], 2015). Prescription pain medications are generally safe for use when taken for a short time and as directed. However, in addition to the relief of pain, they can produce desirable feelings of euphoria that can lead to their misuse.

Because of the rise of opioid-related serious adverse events, such as overdose death, as well as changes in clinical guidelines (Dowell et al., 2016), prescribers have made considerable efforts to decrease the use of long-term opioid medications in recent years (Bohnert et al., 2018). Unfortunately, the use of illegally obtained opioids such as fentanyl and heroin persists, and opioid-related overdose deaths and adverse events continue to be of great concern (CDC, 2019). Although this topic is worthy of extensive examination and intervention, the exclusive focus in this chapter is on those who have been prescribed opioids for pain management by a health care provider.

Usage Descriptions

The terms "misuse," "tolerance," "dependence," and "addiction" are frequently used when discussing opioids, but often there is a lack of understanding or agreement about what these words mean. There is considerable discussion and debate about the best terms for varying phenomena, particularly with regard to prescription opioids (National Center for Injury Prevention and Control, n.d.), and the terminology is often viewed as a gray area. Health care practitioners must be aware of these inconsistencies because they can affect patients' experiences. The brief definitions provided in this chapter reflect the literature and current landscape and are intended to help within the context of this book and in clinical conversations.

Generally, *misuse* is defined as the use of any substance in a manner, situation, amount, or frequency that can cause harm to users or to those around them (U.S. Office of the Surgeon General, 2018). *Prescription opioid misuse* is the use of opioid analgesics in any way other than as directed by a prescribing provider. *Opioid misuse* is frequently used; it is less pejorative and perhaps more desirable because it lacks precision (Manhapra et al., 2018). This can be useful in a gray area, where diagnosis is unclear. Furthermore, the use of terms such as "abuse" or even "opioid use disorder" can engender defensive responses from patients and make communication more difficult. In a study of general practice patients, Von Korff et al. (2011) found opioid misuse—including purposeful oversedation, use of opioid for nonpain purposes, and hoarding or obtaining opioids from multiple sources—to be relatively common. Data from the 2017 National Survey on Drug Use and Health (Center for Behavioral Health Statistics and Quality, 2018) indicate that 11.1 million people aged 12 and older had misused prescription pain relievers in the past year.

Tolerance is a physical process that occurs when a person requires more of a drug to achieve the same effect, something that is commonly experienced with opioids (Morgan & Christie, 2011). A typical clinical scenario is that someone initiates opioids at 5 mg/325 mg of oxycodone/acetaminophen (i.e., Percocet) three times per day with reasonable assistance to pain and function. Over time, their physician increases that to 7.5 mg/325 mg three times per day, and eventually to 10 mg/325 mg four times per day to achieve similar effects. The process of developing tolerance can take months or years, depending on the individual. However, as the dose is increased so is associated risk, and prescribing medical providers typically become concerned with these changes. In addition, escalating the amount of opioids used may increase sensitivity to pain (i.e., hyperalgesia), creating a problem that is not solved with higher doses (Deng et al., 2019). The tolerance process can be very frustrating for patients who feel unable to achieve their initial results and may not understand the hesitance of physicians to increase beyond what are known to be recommended safe doses.

Dependence means that the body has become accustomed to a certain amount of a drug and when that level is lowered or is not available, the person experiences withdrawal (World Health Organization, 2009). Dependence can occur with substances ranging from caffeine and cigarettes to alcohol and opioids. *Withdrawal* is a constellation of uncomfortable physical and psychological symptoms that can range from mild to severe and include but are not limited to nausea or vomiting, sweating, chills, rapid heart rate, headache, agitation (physical and mental), anxiety, increased pain, and disturbed sleep (World Health Organization, 2009). Depending on symptom severity and related distress, when a person is experiencing opioid withdrawal, a medical provider may offer a medication such as clonidine to relieve physical discomfort (Gowing et al., 2016).

The term "opioid addiction," while still used by some, is no longer preferable or part of the fifth edition of the *Diagnostic and Statistical Manual of Mental Disorders* (*DSM-5*; American Psychiatric Association, 2013); it has been replaced by *opioid use disorder* (OUD). This disorder is characterized by impaired social functioning and a loss of control around opioids, including risky use (U.S. Office of the Surgeon General, 2018). The criteria for OUD are outlined in the next section, following a review of important considerations related to chronic opioid use.

Potential Associations With Long-Term Opioid Use

Long-term opioid therapy, also referred to as *chronic opioid therapy*, is defined by the CDC as use of opioids on most days for > 3 months (Dowell et al., 2016). High-risk dosing changed from ≥ 120 mg morphine equivalent dose (MED) to ≥ 90 mg MED, per the 2016 guidelines of the CDC (Dowell et al., 2016). Although opioid-related guidelines provide clear information about the risk factors for use, evidence indicates that the phenomenon of adverse selection is prevalent (Sullivan, 2010): The patients at highest risk of overuse and adverse events receive the highest risk opioid regimens, consisting of high-dose opioid therapy (Edlund et al., 2010; Howe & Sullivan, 2014;

Sullivan, 2010; Sullivan & Howe, 2013). This phenomenon is observed at opioid initiation and in maintenance (Sullivan & Howe, 2013). There are many reasons why this may be the case, though the phenomenon is under-explored in the literature. Possible explanations indicate that more complex psychiatric and social issues can make clinical dynamics more challenging (Frank et al., 2016, 2017). Providers may be compelled to prescribe opioids because of frustration with the lack of improvements, discomfort with unpleasant interactions, or, as identified by Mojtabai (2018), direct-to-consumer pharmaceutical advertising and the campaign to monitor pain as "the fifth vital sign."

Helping patients make informed decisions about opioid use includes sharing information about possible side effects and outcomes. Qualitative interviews suggest that many individuals who take opioids for pain feel that typical media coverage regarding opioid overdose or overuse is not relevant to their situation (Frank et al., 2016). People are often aware that high doses can be dangerous but may be less familiar with other risk factors and potential health impacts of opioids. These key facts about opioids should be shared in a way that is patient-centric and personally meaningful, rather than as a scare tactic that creates defensiveness. Long-term opioid use is linked to various undesirable outcomes, such as

- *poor sleep*: Chronic use of opioid therapy is known to disrupt sleep architecture and sleep stage distribution, disturbances that can cause or contribute to disturbed sleep, fatigue, and daytime sleepiness (Rosen et al., 2019). Opioids are also associated with several types of sleep-disordered breathing, including sleep-related hypoventilation, central sleep apnea, and obstructive sleep apnea. Individuals taking opioids are also more likely to have sleep apnea (Morasco et al., 2014; Rosen et al., 2019).

- *constipation*: Data suggest that 40% to 45% of people using long-term opioids experience constipation (Panchal et al., 2007), which is frequently refractory even with treatment by stool softeners and laxatives (Swegle & Logemann, 2006).

- *poor mood*: Long-term opioid use is associated with various negative mood symptoms, including depression (Scherrer et al., 2016).

- *increased pain*: Chronic opioid therapy can paradoxically induce or sensitize individuals to pain (Lee et al., 2011) and has been associated with lower pain tolerance in nonhuman animal studies and clinical studies with humans (Grant et al., 2007).

- *low testosterone, hypogonadism, sexual dysfunction, and infertility*: Sexual side effects should be discussed so that individuals are aware that they are possible. Because opioids may affect sexual functioning, sexual performance, and health, these potential side effects can hold great importance and may deter individuals from using opioids (Ajo et al., 2016, 2017).

- *nausea*: About 25% of individuals taking long-term opioids experience nausea (Baldini et al., 2012).

Furthermore, many factors increase the risks associated with long-term opioid use (i.e., > 3 months), including

- daily dose over 100 MME (morphine milligram equivalents)
- combination with benzodiazepines (e.g., Klonopin, Valium)
- personal or family history of substance use disorder
- depression
- history of overdose
- age, youthful and elderly (< 30 or > 65)
- respiratory compromise (e.g., sleep apnea; Speed et al., 2018)

Glanz et al. (2018) found nine overdose predictors in a sample of 43,000, and they were validated in a subsequent sample. The predictors included

- age (youthful and elderly)
- mental health diagnosis
- psychotropic prescription
- substance use disorders
- tobacco use
- opioid prescription in year prior to initiating long-term opioids
- daily opioid dose
- hepatitis C
- use of long-acting or extended-release formulation

In addition, various clinical presentations suggest consideration of opioid reduction or discontinuation (U.S. Department of Health and Human Services, 2019b). These include

- pain improvement
- patient interest or request
- absent analgesia
- lack of functional improvement
- aberrant behaviors
- high-risk polypharmacy or medical comorbidities
- side effects that outweigh benefits of medication

Opioid Use Disorder

OUD is a psychological disease that is chronic but treatable (U.S. Office of the Surgeon General, 2018). Evaluating whether someone has OUD and providing the appropriate treatment can literally be a life-saving decision. Before opioid tapering can be considered, a determination regarding OUD must be made, as individuals with the disorder are unlikely to tolerate deprescribing well and are at heightened risk for overdose and seeking other opioids on the street (e.g., heroin).

Although clinical criteria have shifted over time, OUD indicates a problematic use of opioids accompanied by distress and impairments in multiple domains (Dowell et al., 2016). As previously mentioned, the *DSM-5* (American Psychiatric Association, 2013) does not separate opioid abuse and opioid dependence but rather combines them into a single diagnosis of OUD, which is on a continuum including mild (two or three symptoms), moderate (four or five symptoms), and severe (six or more symptoms). To meet the criteria for OUD, an individual must have a problematic pattern of opioid use associated with impairment or distress, as manifested by at least two of the following criteria within a 12-month period:

- taking opioids in larger amounts or over a longer period of time than intended

- a persistent desire or has made unsuccessful efforts to cut down or control opioid use

- spending a great deal of time in activities necessary to obtain the opioid, use the opioid, or recover from its effects

- experiencing cravings or strong urges to use opioids

- failing to fulfill major role obligations at work, school, or home because of recurrent opioid use

- continued opioid use despite persistent or recurrent social or interpersonal problems caused or exacerbated by the effects of opioids

- giving up or reducing important social, occupational, or recreational activities because of opioid use

- engaging in recurrent opioid use in situations in which it is physically hazardous

- continued opioid use despite knowledge that one has a persistent or recurrent physical or psychological problem that is likely to have been caused or exacerbated by opioids

- tolerance, as defined by either (a) a need for markedly increased amounts of opioids to achieve intoxication or the desired effect or (b) markedly diminished effect with continued use of the same amount of an opioid
- withdrawal, as manifested by either (a) the characteristic opioid withdrawal syndrome or (b) taking the same (or a closely related) substance to relieve or avoid withdrawal symptoms

Note, however, that when taking prescribed opioids under appropriate medical supervision, tolerance and withdrawal are not considered criteria for OUD.

These criteria fall into four general categories:

- impaired control (taking more or longer; failed attempts to decrease use; excessive time to obtain; cravings)
- social consequences (not fulfilling social obligations; interpersonal problems; giving up important activities)
- risky use or impacts (use in dangerous situations; physical and psychological problems due to use)
- pharmacologic realities (tolerance or withdrawal)

Determining the presence of OUD is a highly complicated clinical area due to the interplay between prescription opioids, discerning the most accurate diagnoses and treatments, and patients' resistance. The importance and complications of diagnosing and, perhaps more essential, treating OUD appropriately, are discussed further in Chapter 4, along with the details of clinical evaluation.

CONCLUSION

Chronic pain and opioid use are highly complex issues in their own right; when the factors for consideration in defining, evaluating, and treating them are taken together, the complexity increases exponentially. It is beyond the scope of this book to provide an exhaustive background of these related subject areas, but this brief review introduced selected theories, principles, terms, and literature that will assist in providing context to the integrated approaches presented in later chapters.

2 TREATMENT APPROACHES

The Evidence

To optimize all clinical interactions, health care providers must first be familiar with the evidence that supports treatment options and decisions. Recent literature investigating the impacts of behavioral approaches on opioid management is helpful in highlighting the supporting role of these strategies in making medication changes (Darnall et al., 2018; Garland et al., 2020; Sullivan et al., 2017; Zgierska et al., 2016). A recent systematic review and meta-analysis of 60 randomized controlled trials (RCTs) addressing mind–body therapies for opioid-treated pain suggested that these approaches were associated not only with improved pain but also with reduced opioid use (Garland et al., 2020). Finally, it is important for health care professionals to understand the literature regarding the impact of opioid reduction, as sharing the knowledge can significantly allay patient fears. For example, research suggests that for many individuals, long-term pain intensity remains stable or decreases following opioid tapering (Fishbain & Pulikal, 2019; Frank et al., 2017).

https://doi.org/10.1037/0000209-003
Chronic Pain and Opioid Management: Strategies for Integrated Treatment,
by J. L. Murphy and S. Rafie

This chapter includes a review of the expanding body of evidence that supports behavioral health approaches to assist individuals with pain and opioid management. It is critical to note that more research investigating the intersection between pain and opioids is needed, including attempts to understand the neurobiological interactions, psychosocial vulnerabilities, and optimal treatment pathways for this population.

BEHAVIORAL MEDICINE FOR CHRONIC PAIN MANAGEMENT

For those managing chronic pain and opioids, behavioral pain medicine expertise can provide foundational pain education and address concerns about opioid changes. A limited but growing number of studies suggest that concurrent treatment for pain and opioid reductions as well as for opioid use disorders may be both feasible and helpful for patients. In a systematic review, Frank et al. (2017) examined the effectiveness of behavioral interventions in the context of opioid dose reductions. One of the good-quality trials compared a 4-month interactive voice response intervention to usual care among 51 patients with chronic pain (Naylor et al., 2010). Although opioid reduction was an optional goal, participants in the intervention experienced significantly greater reduction in opioids at 4 and 8 months than did those with usual care (Naylor et al., 2010).

Zgierska et al. (2016) did not focus on dose reduction as part of treatment but rather compared an 8-week mindfulness and cognitive behavior-based group with usual care for individuals on long-term opioids. From baseline to 26 weeks, the mean change in daily dose was 10.1 mg morphine equivalent dose (MED) in the treatment group but was only 0.2 mg MED in the control group. Sullivan et al. (2017) addressed opioid reduction as the primary outcome, comparing usual care to a 22-week opioid taper support intervention that involved motivational interviewing and pain self-management education. Both groups had decreased pain severity and opioid dose, and those who received the intervention had significant improvements in pain interference, pain self-efficacy, and perceived opioid problems. In an RCT, Jamison et al. (2010) found that a brief behavioral intervention aided in the management of opioid compliance for patients who were prescribed opioids for chronic back pain and who showed opioid misuse potential.

Barry et al. (2019) evaluated the feasibility and preliminary efficacy of cognitive behavioral therapy (CBT) for opioid use disorder (OUD) and chronic pain, comparing it with standard methadone drug counseling. Attendance, satisfaction, and reduction in pain interference were comparable across groups, and the CBT intervention had higher abstinence rates.

Darnall et al. (2018) examined the impact of a self-help book containing cognitive behavior-based strategies on individuals voluntarily tapering from opioids in a community sample. The study showed a high level of patient engagement, with many individuals voluntarily reducing opioids successfully. However, psychosocial variables remained stable throughout the study, indicating that low-burden behavioral options may be needed to optimize overall outcomes. A number of other studies currently underway (Darnall et al., 2019; Sandhu et al., 2019) are examining the role of behavioral and self-management treatment options on opioid reduction in individuals with chronic pain. The results of these trials will provide valuable information to help determine how we can best provide integrated pain and opioid management.

Data across pain treatments indicate that psychosocial factors strongly influence chronic pain treatment outcomes (Edwards, Dworkin, et al., 2016). Despite this and the ample evidence demonstrating the effectiveness of behavioral health modalities in improved pain functioning (Chou et al., 2016; Darnall, 2018; Ehde et al., 2014; Schütze et al., 2018; Stewart et al., 2015), often these treatments are still considered a last resort or are reserved for individuals with more significant mental health issues. Evidence over the last century indicates that pain is not solely physical or sensory—it is an integrated experience that is affected by various cognitive, affective, social, and environmental factors. Pain is a complex process and therefore requires treatment that attends to all parts of the equation.

Many behavioral medicine options are available for individuals with pain; however, the breadth and depth of research is so robust that only those treatments used most routinely and effectively are reviewed in this chapter. Some of the selected studies target a particular pain location, such as low back or fibromyalgia. Others target a broader category, such as musculoskeletal pain, and systematic reviews are generally inclusive across pain locations and conditions.

Cognitive Behavioral Therapy

The evidence for effectiveness in treating individuals with chronic pain is strongest for CBT; it is, therefore, considered the gold standard psychological intervention for the treatment of chronic pain (Eccleston et al., 2013; Ehde et al., 2014; Morley et al., 1999; Skelly et al., 2018; Williams et al., 2012). It is the longest standing, it is employed most routinely, and it has the most broad-based support for efficacy for application across pain conditions, from migraines to multiple sclerosis to cancer.

CBT for chronic pain (CBT-CP) highlights the central role and interaction between cognitive, behavioral, and emotional factors in the experience of chronic pain. The experience of pain is influenced by cognitive and affective processes, and an individual's thoughts and feelings can impact pain intensity, level of disability, mood, and activity engagement. Extensive scientific investigation solidifies the important reasons for using CBT-CP to address the behaviors and mindset that affect pain and have a positive impact on pain-related functioning (Knoerl et al., 2016).

Studies provide evidence for the effectiveness of CBT-CP in patient outcomes, reflecting improvements in pain intensity, cognitions such as pain-related catastrophizing, physical functioning, coping skills, and self-efficacy (Darnall, 2018; Ehde et al., 2014; Schütze et al., 2018; Stewart et al., 2015). A 2012 Cochrane review that included 4,788 participants (Williams et al., 2012) is the most stringent analysis to date of psychological therapies for chronic pain. The review included only treatments that were behavioral or cognitive behavioral in nature, as other options, such as those that were acceptance-based, did not meet the preliminary criteria for scientific rigor. CBT showed effects on pain and functioning comparable to standard medical care for pain. CBT for chronic pain, compared with usual treatment and wait list controls, had moderate effects on mood and catastrophizing and small effects on pain and disability at treatment conclusion. Behavioral treatments had no significant effects in these areas.

CBT was also found to be an effective treatment for reducing highly anxious thinking about pain and anticipating future pain. Richmond et al. (2015) reviewed RCTs that included 3,359 participants who had nonspecific chronic low back pain. They found that CBT yielded moderate to large effects for pain and disability in both the short term and the long term, as compared with guideline-based active treatments.

The Agency for Healthcare Research and Quality (Skelly et al., 2018) conducted a review to assess which noninvasive, nonpharmacological treatments for common chronic pain conditions (i.e., chronic low back and neck pain, fibromyalgia, osteoarthritis, chronic tension headache) improved pain and function for at least 1 month posttreatment. The psychological therapies included CBT, biofeedback, relaxation techniques, and acceptance and commitment therapy. While researchers found a moderate strength of evidence for psychological therapies on the whole, when individual approaches were compared, CBT was most consistently associated with pain-related improvements. Particularly when used to address chronic LBP and fibromyalgia, CBT improved pain and function in the short, intermediate, and long term, above any other nonpharmacological treatment options reviewed. Results from neuropathic pain trials were inconclusive in the analysis of CBT or group psychotherapy efficacy (Eccleston et al., 2015); however, many studies support the use of CBT for a range of chronic pain conditions in adult and pediatric populations (Eccleston & Crombez, 2017).

Acceptance and Commitment Therapy

Acceptance and commitment therapy (ACT) emphasizes increasing psychological flexibility through acceptance of thoughts and feelings, attending to the present, and focusing on personal values. While it is a cognitive and behavioral therapy, ACT differs from traditional CBT for pain in its lack of focus on challenging and changing unhelpful thoughts (Dahl & Lundgren, 2006; McCracken & Vowles, 2014; Vowles & McCracken, 2008). For those who may be fixated on getting rid of pain entirely, as many are, ACT addresses the hopelessness that arises from trying to control things that cannot be controlled. The aim is to increase acceptance of pain and decrease the impact of pain-related thoughts and emotions by establishing improved patterns of behavioral performance. Specifically, increasing identification and engagement in valued activities shifts the focus to a meaningful life and encourages flexible thinking and commitment.

ACT has been well studied and is a strong behavioral medicine option for pain. A 2011 systematic review and meta-analysis of acceptance-based interventions for pain found small effect sizes for reduction of pain intensity and depression and small to moderate effect sizes for mental and physical health (Vcchof et al., 2011). Haun and McCracken's (2014) systematic review of chronic pain found that ACT primarily enhanced physical function and decreased distress compared with inactive treatments.

A more recent study (Gilpin et al., 2017) found that ACT assists in increasing pain acceptance, which is associated with improvements in mood, avoidance, and disability. A systematic review of 11 trials that included ACT for chronic pain (Hughes et al., 2017) found small to medium effects for functioning, anxiety, and depression. Medium to large effects were found for measures of pain acceptance and psychological flexibility, which ACT specifically targets. No significant improvements were found for pain intensity or quality of life across studies.

A growing literature strongly suggests that ACT is effective in treating chronic pain and can assist those with chronic pain in achieving personal goals and improving quality of life. ACT has shown efficacy as a clinical intervention for individuals with musculoskeletal pain (e.g., low back, neck) and whiplash-related disorders (Sturgeon, 2014). It has also shown promise as an accompaniment to physiotherapy for improving treatment outcomes; this use for ACT is currently under further study.

Mindfulness-Based Interventions

Mindfulness-based interventions (e.g., mindfulness-based stress reduction [MBSR], mindfulness-based cognitive therapy [MBCT], mindfulness-oriented recovery enhancement [MORE]) are increasingly available as empirically supported behavioral treatment options for chronic pain. These treatment options are characterized by attention to the present moment with openness, curiosity, and acceptance (Hilton et al., 2017). The language of mindfulness has assumed a more prominent position in popular culture because of the de-emphasis of analgesics such as opioids for pain. This change has led patients to inquire more frequently about options that incorporate meditation.

A variety of studies have examined the impact of mindfulness on specific pain conditions (e.g., low back pain, fibromyalgia), and comprehensive reviews of RCTs have been published (Bawa et al., 2015; Cramer et al., 2012; Lauche et al., 2013; Reiner et al., 2013). Improvements have been noted in depressive symptoms and coping, and small positive effects have been shown for reduction in pain (Bawa et al., 2015; Cramer et al., 2012; Hilton et al., 2017). Hilton and colleagues' (2017) systematic review and meta-analysis of mindfulness meditation RCTs showed statistically significant improvements associated with a small decrease in pain intensity (low-quality evidence), physical health–related quality of life (low-quality evidence), mental health–related quality of life (moderate-quality evidence), and depression symptoms (high-quality evidence) compared with treatment as usual, passive controls, and education or support groups.

Chiesa and Serretti (2011) reviewed six RCTs and four controlled trials of MBSR and closely derived mind–body interventions for chronic pain and found mixed results. Of the seven studies that included pain intensity measures, three found that mindfulness was better than a wait-list control, one suggested it was better than an educational group but less efficacious than a CBT group, and one suggested it was better than progressive muscle relaxation. Other studies did not note any significant difference between mindfulness plus qigong compared with an educational support group or between mindfulness plus massage as compared with a wait list. Chiesa and Serretti concluded that the evidence was not sufficient to determine whether mindfulness-based interventions could be more efficacious than nonspecific interventions such as support and educational control groups for the reduction of pain and depressive symptoms in patients with chronic pain.

As defined by Kabat-Zinn (1982, 1990, 2003), MBSR has a well-defined protocol. It involves an outpatient program that combines meditation, body awareness, and yoga to increase self-regulation and improve management of the chronic pain experience (Kabat-Zinn, 1982). A single large RCT (Morone et al., 2016) suggested that MBSR was effective for low back pain, but this study was limited by its focus only on a population of older adults. An additional RCT that compared MBSR with treatment as usual and with CBT for pain (Cherkin et al., 2016) stands out due to its methodological quality: For those with chronic low back pain, MBSR was as effective as CBT, and more effective than usual care, for clinically meaningful improvement in back pain and associated functional limitations as well as pain bother-someness. Across reviews, authors consistently express that the evidence for mindfulness interventions is limited due to methodological issues that raise concerns (e.g., lack of intent-to-treat analysis, low follow-up rate, small samples, inadequately powered studies) and advocate that higher quality studies should be conducted prior to making strong recommendations.

Relaxation and Biofeedback

Stress is generally recognized as a key factor in the chronic pain process (Melzack, 1999). Because stress plays a role in exacerbating and maintaining pain, managing and reducing physical and emotional tension are typically integral parts of chronic pain treatment. The effectiveness of relaxation techniques to address stress and manage both acute and chronic pain conditions has been determined across the literature (Carroll & Seers, 1998). Through various approaches, patients learn to gain awareness of physiological and psychological states and reduce tension levels by triggering the relaxation response through activation of the parasympathetic nervous system (Benson et al., 1974). Common relaxation techniques applied to chronic pain include but are not limited to diaphragmatic breathing, progressive muscle relaxation, visualization, guided imagery, autogenic training, and body scan; the application of these strategies to pain and opioid management is explored in subsequent chapters. With a better understanding of how physiological responses can affect pain, individuals can learn to quiet unwanted responses.

Biofeedback is a technique by which patients learn to monitor and regulate physiological cues using the information provided by external feedback (Yucha & Montgomery, 2008). Individuals are connected to measurement instruments that rapidly provide data regarding skin temperature, heart rate, muscle activity, respiration, and other physiological functions. This technique allows patients to better understand their own responses and to exercise self-regulatory control over processes that have often become automatic and unhelpful in the pain experience. Robust evidence suggests that biofeedback is effective as part of migraine treatment; for other pain conditions, it is typically most effective when used in conjunction with other cognitive behavioral approaches (Yucha & Montgomery, 2008). Both relaxation and biofeedback can be offered on their own but are frequently incorporated into other forms of behavioral treatments such as CBT or ACT.

Motivational Interviewing

Motivational interviewing (MI) is an evidence-based intervention and style of collaborative communication that can effectively facilitate communication between patient and provider. The literature for MI, as applied to those with chronic pain, is mixed, and more trials are needed. A meta-analysis and systematic review of its impacts on those with chronic pain (Alperstein & Sharpe, 2016) suggested that patients indicated a small to moderate overall effect in adherence from baseline to treatment completion but not at follow-up. Short-term effects for pain intensity were not maintained, and studies were insufficient to determine impacts on physical functioning.

Studies combining MI with exercise have found varying effects. An RCT of those with fibromyalgia (Ang et al., 2013) focused on whether MI or self-management increased engagement in an exercise program. This study suggested that, despite a lack of significant differences between groups at 6-month follow-up, individuals in the MI group had more benefit in walking and physical activity in the short term than those in the self-management group. Another study (Tse et al., 2013) found that older adults in an integrated 8-week exercise and MI program had significant improvements in pain self-efficacy, anxiety, mobility, and quality of life in comparison with those in usual care.

In a study of individuals with various forms of cancer pain (Thomas et al., 2012), those randomly assigned to a group that received MI-based coaching sessions plus education reported significantly more improvement in pain-related interference, general health, mental health, and vitality than those receiving education only or usual care; however, attitudinal barrier scores were not different for the groups across time points. An RCT of individuals with knee osteoarthritis (KOA) and rheumatoid arthritis (RA; Gilbert et al., 2018) compared people who received brief physician recommendations to increase physical activity with people who received the same guidance and MI over a year of treatment. The individuals with KOA experienced modest improvement in self-reported function and pain, compared with the control group, but they experienced no significant improvements in physical activity. For individuals with RA, no significant intervention effects were found.

Catastrophizing and Expectations

Pain catastrophizing refers to a negative cognitive and affective mental state related to actual or anticipated pain experiences (Sullivan et al., 2001). It is a construct characterized by pain rumination or focus, the magnification of pain-related negative effects, and feelings of pain-related hopelessness (Sullivan et al., 1995). High levels of catastrophizing are associated with depression and anxiety (Sullivan et al., 1995) and poorer medical outcomes (Mankovsky et al., 2012). One study (Toth et al., 2014) found that catastrophizing had a maladaptive effect on pharmacotherapy for neuropathic pain, with higher catastrophizing levels associated with poorer pain relief and greater likelihood of discontinuing pharmacotherapy. Research also indicates a relationship between pain catastrophizing and heightened reported pain intensity (Flor et al., 1993; Sullivan et al., 1995). Brain imaging scans show that individuals who engage in higher levels of catastrophizing activate areas of the brain associated with pain processing (Seminowicz & Davis, 2006; Seminowicz et al., 2013). On a positive note, research indicates that behavioral treatment options such as CBT are effective for lowering levels of pain catastrophizing (Schütze et al., 2018; Stewart et al., 2015). By understanding the literature on pain-related catastrophizing, health care providers can better explain the powerful role of thoughts in the pain experience and motivate people to adapt through treatment.

While catastrophizing is a cognitive process characterized by the expectation of a negative outcome, general expectations regarding pain and pain treatment are important mediational factors in pain outcomes and are often overlooked when considering treatment approaches (Roditi & Robinson, 2011). The placebo literature indicates that expectations are a crucial component of treatment, resulting in measurable changes in pain perception that is self-reported but also confirmed at the neurobiological level (Roditi & Robinson, 2011; Wager et al., 2004). However, as Fields (2018) astutely noted, it would be more accurate to acknowledge that every pain treatment has an expectation component that plays a key role in how it is received. An analysis of four acupuncture RCTs that compared chronic pain treatment with sham intervention (Linde et al., 2007) showed that individuals with higher outcome expectations also showed greater improvement. Similarly, an analysis of approximately 600 patients engaged in chiropractic care (Eklund et al., 2019) found that individuals with a high expectation of improvement were 58% more likely to report improvement at a subsequent visit, a finding that was not mediated by factors such as pain intensity or psychological profile.

Although the extensive literature on expectations is beyond the scope of this review, it is clinically important to note that in persistent conditions such as chronic pain, early treatment "failures" will lead to an expectation of more unsuccessful treatments (Fields, 2018). That this can become a self-fulfilling prophecy suggests the critical importance of both providing education about the complex nature of chronic pain and establishing realistic expectations for treatment outcomes as early as possible. Furthermore, this also supports the need to share evidence regarding the role of behavioral interventions for pain as soon as possible because patient preference and expectations may interfere with engagement and outcomes (Beasley et al., 2017; Bee et al., 2016). The MUSICAL study (Bee et al., 2016), which focused on perspectives for treatment delivery among those with chronic widespread pain, found that psychological therapy had connotations of stigma and social judgment, whereas an option such as physical therapy was far more acceptable due to its support of a mechanistic issue. On a positive note, this study also showed that the experience of psychological intervention often exceeded expectations and led to physical and emotional benefits.

PSYCHOLOGICAL FACTORS AND OPIOID MISUSE

Those with chronic pain and co-occurring mental health disorders are at higher risk for misuse of prescribed opioids (Chou et al., 2009; Manchikanti et al., 2007; Turk et al., 2008; van Rijswijk et al., 2019; Wasan et al., 2007). Wasan et al. (2015) found that individuals with high negative affect achieved only about half of the analgesic effect observed in those with low negative affect. In a study of patients with musculoskeletal pain, Martel et al. (2013) demonstrated that pain-related catastrophizing was a unique predictor for opioid misuse. Arteta and colleagues (2016) found that catastrophizing, anxiety, and depression predicted higher risk for prescription opioid misuse; other studies have also indicated that individuals with higher levels of depression are at increased risk for opioid misuse (Feingold et al., 2018). Furthermore, individuals with psychiatric comorbidities and high levels of distress appear to have brain-based changes in pain modulation that may contribute to decreased benefit from opioid treatment and set the stage for the need for higher dosing (Edwards, Dolman, et al., 2016). McHugh and colleagues (2016) found that distress intolerance was associated with opioid misuse in individuals with chronic pain who were also prescribed opioids. This factor can be impacted and modified through the use of behavioral pain medicine, which may mitigate risk. Hruschak et al.'s (2018) review of the literature regarding individuals with chronic pain and OUD reinforced the potential utility of psychosocial interventions such as CBT, ACT, and mindfulness for this population, while noting the dearth of empirical data and need for further research.

OPIOID REDUCTION: WHAT THE LITERATURE SUGGESTS

The literature regarding the role and impacts of behavioral treatments on opioid tapering is limited but growing, as there is a keen interest in expanding research in this area. In general, strong evidence for the efficacy of any treatment options in opioid deprescribing for individuals with chronic pain is lacking, primarily due to the scarcity of RCTs investigating interventions in this population (Eccleston et al., 2017). This is therefore a topic that demands increased research attention.

An important recent systematic review and meta-analysis of mind–body therapies for opioid-treated pain (Garland et al., 2020) included 60 RCTs with 6,404 patients. Garland et al. (2020) found that these approaches—CBT, relaxation, meditation, hypnosis, guided imagery, and therapeutic suggestion—were associated with moderate improvements in pain and small reductions in opioid use. Of note, although most studies including meditation, CBT, and hypnosis found improved opioid-related outcomes, studies involving relaxation, guided imagery, and suggestion showed less improvement. As noted in the 2017 Cochrane review (Eccleston et al., 2017), numerous nonrandomized studies were not included but showed major opioid reductions in the context of intensive rehabilitation treatment milieus that included a variety of behavioral and physical modalities.

Despite the lack of evidence for outcomes, the literature and clinical experiences of patients and providers suggest a fear of making changes in opioid medications for individuals with chronic pain. At times, individuals with pain want to decrease opioid use because they experience negative side effects such as sedation and constipation, lack of significant functional benefit, and unease with feeling overly reliant on medication. Increasingly, prescribers encourage patients to reduce opioid dosages because of safety concerns, but reducing opioids can be a daunting proposition when an individual is in pain. Behavioral medicine can play an especially helpful role in both decreasing concerns and increasing strategies for management.

Qualitative studies have helped to shed light on the perspectives of both patients and prescribers regarding reducing opioid use (Frank et al., 2016; Toye et al., 2017). A qualitative evidence synthesis of health care providers' experiences prescribing opioids (Toye et al., 2017) revealed several common themes, including uncertainty about when to prescribe, a default assumption that the primary aim is to relieve pain, and attempts to determine who had "real" or "legitimate" pain, often based on nonclinical factors and gut feelings. Frank et al. (2016) described patient attitudes about the continuum of tapering (i.e., not tapering, tapering, completed tapering). The study uncovered the following themes: low perceived risk of overdose, emphasis on pain relief now rather than concern about future adverse impacts, pessimism about nonopioid pharmacological and nonpharmacological options for pain management, fear of increased pain, and fear of opioid withdrawal. In this sample, individuals who had tapered reported improved quality of life after shedding unwanted side effects and endorsed similar pain levels (Frank et al., 2016). Henry et al. (2019) conducted patient interviews (i.e., focus group, individual) to clarify patient experiences with opioid tapering and developed a conceptual framework to assist clinicians. Themes that surfaced were patient perceptions of fluctuating pain and opioid needs, the effort across domains required to taper opioids, and personal strategies to manage the tapering process (e.g., keeping a just-in-case supply of opioids).

Trials indicating the effects of opioid reduction suggest that many common patient fears are not supported by data. The most significant patient fear is increased pain due to decreased prescribing or discontinuation of opioid analgesics, but the data do not support this outcome, as pain tends to remain stable or even decrease (Murphy et al., 2013). Fishbain and Pulikal (2019) conducted an evidence-based systematic review to determine changes that occurred at taper completion, defined as no longer using opioid analgesics for pain management. In these studies that included over 2,100 individuals with chronic pain combined, 80% reported pain had improved at the conclusion of tapering, and 15% reported that it remained the same (i.e., did not increase). Frank et al. (2017) conducted a systematic review of outcomes related to various strategies for opioid dose reduction or discontinuation that occurred in contexts ranging from interdisciplinary pain programs to outpatient options. While the majority of studies were of poor quality methodologically, all studies of fair quality found improved pain after opioid deprescribing. Furthermore, all studies found improvements in quality of life and functioning after tapering.

CONCLUSION

For health care providers to best assist individuals contending with pain and opioid-related issues, it is essential first to understand the empirical support surrounding the treatment options. Adequate patient education about the science of behavioral medicine is a critical element of facilitating buy-in for treatment, which, as discussed, is particularly important for individuals who have what are often believed to be purely physical conditions. Understanding the evidence can help strengthen the case for why integration of these strategies is not only beneficial but critical for optimal outcomes. A breadth of research on available treatments suggests that all share the common goals of helping individuals improve their functioning and quality of life. Each emphasizes recovery, engagement, and personal empowerment. These approaches should be used when indicated for patients struggling with management of their pain and opioids.

3 THE PATIENT–PROVIDER RELATIONSHIP

The patient–provider relationship is a central factor influencing the success of treatment in both general medicine and psychotherapy settings (Hall et al., 2010). The alliance between patient and provider has been extensively studied as determining treatment outcomes and must be a priority for providers approaching this population (Kelley et al., 2014). Understanding dynamics that support patient growth will allow health care providers to approach treatment more effectively. Numerous factors have been identified as critical for progress in patients, such as communication (Ha & Longnecker, 2010) and setting expectations (Penney et al., 2017; Wampold, 2015). Especially important in relationships with patients who experience chronic pain and are on opioid therapy is trust in their provider (Sherman et al., 2018). Given a population with a potentially turbulent history with the health care system, providers must remain mindful of language choices and maintain a sensitive approach throughout treatment. This chapter explains why the patient–provider relationship is so important and addresses the components that lead to a successful relationship.

https://doi.org/10.1037/0000209-004
Chronic Pain and Opioid Management: Strategies for Integrated Treatment,
by J. L. Murphy and S. Rafie

THE IMPORTANCE OF THE PATIENT'S EXPERIENCE

Individuals with chronic pain who use opioids often feel they are not heard, not believed, or both (Upshur et al., 2010). The emotional reactions these individuals feel toward their health care providers reflect their accumulated prior experiences, many of which may have been negative. As they go through numerous evaluations, procedures, and therapies, they encounter a wide variety of practitioners, from pain specialists to generalists, primary care physicians to substance use counselors. Each encounter presents the possibility of an unpleasant interaction, inconsistent explanations for their symptoms, shaming inquiries, or conflicting treatment plans (Esquibel & Borkan, 2014). And as the literature suggests, entering into encounters with these expectations does not provide positive scaffolding (Fields, 2018). The compounding effect results in patients often feeling frustrated, mistrustful, and hopeless regarding improvement.

As providers obtain individuals' medical backgrounds and current functioning, they begin to understand the journey and can empathize with the patients' concerns. It is not uncommon for the first emotion conveyed in treatment to be one of mistrust, particularly if the patient feels that they were sent by their prescribing physician so that they might change their opioid regimen (Upshur et al., 2010). In this case, aligning with patients so they feel understood will reduce their defensiveness. For example, conveying interest in the patient's personal health goals and apologizing for insensitivity faced in certain settings can be helpful. The mistrust may stem from lack of overall treatment progress or inconsistent messaging from providers, and a new provider can offer support and validate the patient's feelings, which are likely to include distress and exhaustion.

Despite the potential benefits of various treatments, patients often struggle with the prolonged trajectory. The time since their initial injury or onset of pain varies, as do previous treatments. Prior work-up and treatments may have included multiple medication trials, physical therapy, aquatic therapy, acupuncture, various injections and interventional procedures, aquatic therapy, chiropractic care, or surgery. Each step may require new referrals, waiting for evaluation appointments, waiting for results, insurance authorization, scheduling far in advance, the stress and pain of undergoing treatment, and sometimes recovery from the treatment itself. It may also feel exhausting to share their story of pain and opioids with so many people in multiple settings. The process may take a toll on the person's mood, relationships, and sleep (Nicassio & Wallston, 1992; Strunin & Boden, 2004).

PROVIDER CHARACTERISTICS THAT SUPPORT A GOOD RELATIONSHIP

The health care provider's role is to initiate and maintain a supportive and helpful tone in all interactions. No matter the discipline, the relationship thrives when the provider is respectful, caring, and understanding. While some patients will present with challenging issues and interpersonal styles, the response is to return to a set of key principles that will guide treatment. This approach combines basic clinical skills and those tailored for patients with pain and opioids, creating a dynamic approach that facilitates positive patient choices.

For health care providers, the use of the general foundational principles for helping others—active listening, empathy, and provision of support—is the best place to start when considering rapport building. Carl Rogers (1946), the father of person-centered therapy, described the core conditions for therapeutic change as warmth, understanding, safety, and acceptance. These principles can be extended to characteristics that facilitate the course of behavioral medicine and beyond. Because so many patients enter the clinical scenario with prior negative experiences as well as some skepticism or uncertainty regarding behavioral treatment in general, the following foundation sets the stage for a positive clinical dynamic.

The Basics

Warmth is a key characteristic of clinicians that allows the patient to feel immediately comfortable in treatment. Simple gestures and the use of nonverbal communication, such as smiling, speaking with a friendly tone, and even offering tissues, convey a sense of warmth and caring. Studies show patients are satisfied with care when they perceive providers are listening to their concerns, empathize, and take time for patients (Ha & Longnecker, 2010). The provider can literally "welcome" the patient to treatment and introduce themselves by name, title, and role on the treatment team. Then, the provider can acknowledge the possible defenses that are commonly voiced by patients, such as doubts or fears caused by stigma associated with exploring behavioral treatment options or perhaps concerns about speaking to an allied health provider about opioid medications and pain. This introduction conveys understanding that engaging in behavioral interventions may be a difficult step. An introduction of this sort sets the stage for reduced defensiveness in the patient and improved communication. The relationship thrives when the provider is supportive and respectful.

Understanding the patient's perspective is critical in relationship building, particularly regarding the patient's stance on medication changes. This part of relationship building takes many forms, from being fully present and listening actively to being compassionate and empathic. However, the provider must have an accurate empathic understanding of the person's subjective world (Bandura, 1977, 1982), which requires engaging in open-ended discussion rather than making assumptions about their experience. The provider can demonstrate compassion by acknowledging that the patient completed numerous treatments that may not have worked or may have left them still challenged by their pain. Another common scenario is that the person previously tried to cease or reduce opioid use but was unsuccessful. Their previous attempts at behavioral change can lead to development of a powerful narrative and an important exploration of the person's motivations, the factors that supported the change, and potential obstacles. Evidence supports individualized treatment plans created with patients dealing with chronic pain, especially when the provider takes the patient's values and barriers into consideration (Harman et al., 2014). Furthermore, by informing the patient of the key areas that will be discussed throughout treatment, such as experiences with opioids and pain's impact on sleep, mood, and relationships, the provider conveys an accurate understanding of the challenges patients face. Providers must also take into consideration sensitivity to cultural differences (Campbell & Edwards, 2012; Murphy et al., 2016; Santoro & Santoro, 2018).

Trust between patient and provider is necessary to do the work, and it is an important component of the patient–provider relationship among patients with chronic pain who are on chronic opioid therapy (Sherman et al., 2018). Studies show that trust enhances the therapeutic alliance in physical rehabilitation for chronic musculoskeletal pain (Kinney et al., 2018). Trust begins to develop during initial interactions, based on the clinician's demonstrated warmth and understanding, and grows throughout the course of treatment. For this reason, establishing open communication and trust is critical to building a therapeutic alliance in the rehabilitation setting (Bunzli et al., 2016; Harman et al., 2014). Providers should be genuine in their communication with patients and should collaborate to find a direction that reflects both the patient's personal objectives and the clinical recommendations. If the patient returns to a visit reporting difficulty adhering to the agreed-upon goal for the week, the provider should remain nonjudgmental and should maintain an air of safety in the room so that the patient can honestly report their experiences, good or bad. This non-judgmental approach comes from unconditional acceptance of the patient.

Of course, there will be boundaries and limits; however, if expectations and treatment goals are clearly defined, then progress is more likely (Wampold, 2015). A nonjudgmental health care professional will help problem-solve with the patient until they reach a realistic goal, taking into account the emotional, social, and health factors that impact tapering.

Next-Level Dynamics

The foundation of a warm, understanding, and trusting patient–provider relationship allows people to lower their defenses and use treatment as an opportunity for functional improvement and reduced reliance on opioids as the primary strategy for pain management. The focus then shifts to moving patients forward toward their goals of increased use of wellness-focused self-management strategies for chronic pain and opioid management. Through provision of psychoeducation, skills training, and practicing these approaches in the real world, the patient gains insight into unhelpful behaviors and cognitions as well as a set of alternatives for pain management. This process is collaborative, wherein the patient and provider review the successes and challenges as strategies and skills are implemented at home.

Problem-solving is a useful strategy that not only facilitates action planning but also enhances the therapeutic rapport. It is well established as an effective intervention for reducing mental and physical health problems (Malouff et al., 2007). This intervention is typically used to troubleshoot a setback or a goal that was not achieved. Reframing failures as miscalculations will allow the person to understand the problem more easily and to focus on identifying solutions. The provider can use these conversations to facilitate and fine-tune the patient's understanding of pain management skills, such as activity pacing, and to develop realistic and achievable goals together. These conversations are best approached compassionately; the conversation demonstrates that self-compassion is necessary for living well with chronic pain.

Feedback regarding strengths and achievements should be regularly provided by the health care provider, with an emphasis on the person's use of certain skills to generate outcomes. This feedback boosts self-efficacy, which is a significant correlate of outcomes in treatment for chronic pain (Jackson et al., 2014). For example, if a patient reports increased socialization, the provider can encourage the patient to consider what led to the change and how they felt as a result. Usually, this reflection conjures positive emotional associations, such as feeling satisfied with their accomplishment or feeling "like myself again." Providers should take this occasion to be present with the emotion in the room and reflect back the efforts made to achieve those results. Encouragement and positive reinforcement are generally appreciated and further support the patient–provider relationship.

Modeling is an exceptionally useful tool for building a person's sense of self-efficacy when they are struggling to activate or make change. Patients learn through their own experiences as well as by seeing others successfully attempt activities that they see as threatening, thus vicariously facing the fear and boosting self-efficacy (Bandura, 1977). Studies of populations undergoing pain rehabilitation benefit similarly from both individual and group treatments (Rose et al., 1997). The group dynamic can be a powerful force that demonstrates the universality of the condition and can provide an individual a vicarious experience. Modeling occurs through observing peers overcoming obstacles as well as through normalization of fears by the provider.

SEEING BOTH SIDES

Instead of conceptualizing patients and providers on different sides of an issue, as is sometimes the default setting for those with pain, practitioners should consider the common ground between them. This approach can draw people together, rather than highlighting the divisiveness that is seen far too often. Several areas of shared experience exist between patients and providers, such as feeling frustrated and sometimes exhausted with their side of the pain experience.

Table 3.1 provides examples of how the patient and provider may view the same topics differently. Openly discussing topics such as these can help decrease the tense nature that can be part of some clinical interactions.

TABLE 3.1. Patient and Provider Challenges

Patient	Provider
Numerous unsuccessful treatments with perceived lack of improvement	Numerous unsuccessful treatments with reported lack of improvement
Unknowns regarding cause or diagnosis	Unknowns regarding cause or diagnosis
Uncertainty regarding whether the pain is believed	Uncertainty regarding whether the pain should be believed
Having the desire for help but feeling nothing else can be done	Having the desire to help but feeling little else can be done
Do they think I am exaggerating?	Are they exaggerating?

If individuals with pain and the people caring for them are comfortable discussing challenges, they are apt to see that they both want the patient to feel better and both feel disheartened about the lack of progress, instead of being on opposing sides. The inclusion of behavioral interventions can be helpful to provide validation and can be helpful for sharing information about the limitations of the biomedical approach, expectations for outcomes, and the role of self-management in improving pain and opioid management.

BUILDING THE RELATIONSHIP WHEN THE PATIENT IS ANGRY

The collaborative clinician creates a trusting and therapeutic treatment environment, in which most patients feel safe to disclose their struggle with pain and opioids. However, this is not always the case, despite best efforts from providers. The patient–provider relationship can be challenging when patients arrive to treatment with accumulated prior negative experiences that can leave them angry and resentful toward all health care providers, regardless of the provider's motivations. Sometimes this frustration is expressed generally, but other times it is directed at the provider, particularly when a patient is displeased with the responses they receive, no matter how well reasoned. The reality is that in a typical health care interaction, there are two people in the room who are both human. It is understandable that the provider also has reactions to the experience, particularly when it is provocative or emotionally charged. However, the provider can build a better relationship with the patient by responding appropriately, which includes managing their own reactions. Strategies include the following:

- *Staying in control of interactions with all patients*, even those who are more likely to elicit resistance and negative emotions.

- *Monitoring and managing distress by increasing awareness and using tools to stay grounded.* For example, the provider might say to the patient, "Observe your internal state throughout the experience. What state were you in when you entered the room? Are you escalating, becoming agitated, or using shallow breathing?" The provider might then recommend that the patient use mini deep breathing to gain physical and mental balance: "Take a deep breath in for a count of six, and then take a deep breath out to a count of six. Breathe out tension and toxicity. This type of breathing can be done before you enter the room or more briefly, even one pause for breath, during the exchange."

- *Being aware of parallel process.* This process, wherein the health care provider recreates or "parallels" the patient's experience, can be harmful. Providers should avoid mirroring the patient's negative emotional state or being provoked by emotionally charged statements. Emotions are contagious. If a provider is calm, collected, and positive, it is more difficult for patients to maintain anger and frustration.

- *Steering the conversation by staying focused on the present and what can be done now to help the patient.*

- *Routinely evaluating the effectiveness of the treatment.* Is the treatment therapeutic? If a patient continues to resist committing fully, it may not be the right time to engage.

CONCLUSION

The patient–provider relationship is one that can be fraught with challenges or nurtured for a successful partnership. Together, the patient and provider can form a therapeutic alliance and can improve the outcomes derived from treatment. Certain traits within the provider support this approach, such as warmth, understanding, and trust, which are the foundation for open communication, listening, and empathy. However, additional clinical skills of the provider—such as problem-solving interventions, providing feedback, and modeling—are equally important. Throughout each encounter with patients managing both pain and opioids, the provider must remember to engage in patient-centered care, engaging the patient in collaborative discussions regarding treatment goals and plans that incorporate their values and barriers. Patients may be understandably angry, exhausted, depressed, or some combination, resulting from their experience and struggle living with persistent pain. Providers play an important role in creating a supportive environment in which patients may grow toward a healthier next step.

II PHASE 1: PREPARING FOR CHANGE

The beginning is the most important part of the work.

—Plato

INTRODUCTION

As with many other chronic health conditions, considering behavioral changes can be challenging no matter what the motivator (Kelly & Barker, 2016). Hesitation, ambivalence, and resistance are expected parts of the process for those who contend with pain and opioid issues. The preference toward more provider-driven treatments that require less patient involvement, such as medications or even massage, is understandable—these options can provide benefits while requiring limited individual effort or introspection. On the other hand, engaging in a collaborative treatment that addresses all aspects of the pain and opioid experience can be a daunting proposition, charged with many sources of resistance. Individuals with pain may not want to engage in self-managed strategies if they believe that a medical solution to eliminate their pain is still possible. For those who have felt accused of drug seeking or being opioid focused, treatment engagement may be viewed as confessing to a problem that is inaccurate or incomplete. Those who struggle with pain and opioids, as well as some providers, may see participating in behavioral treatments as a failure. One aim of this book is to change that belief.

It is critical at the start of treatment to explore patients' experiences and history, including their current concerns about and expectations for pain care and opioid use. Health care providers must carefully and comprehensively evaluate the biopsychosocial factors that impact the individual experience (Turk & Robinson, 2011). Although the purpose of this step is to understand individuals better and prepare them for treatment concepts and strategies, the clinical reality is that patients may never feel fully prepared or motivated. This feeling is common and should be normalized for individuals struggling with pain and opioid management. They have likely tried many different treatment options, each with limited lasting benefit, and therefore may feel dubious about any other offerings. In these instances, forge ahead when the patient is willing—it is difficult, if not impossible, to predict who will succeed with behavioral treatment strategies. The first step is indeed the hardest, and individuals should be supported in this process and applauded for considering a whole-person approach that takes their complexities into consideration. A provider who takes the opportunity to collaboratively discuss concerns about deprescribing may also offer the patient reassurance and confidence to initiate or maintain opioid changes. The foundational work at this stage will help individualize care and may prime people who struggle with pain and opioids for the best possible outcome moving forward.

4 EVALUATE THE PATIENT'S FUNCTIONING AND WELL-BEING

Individuals who present with chronic pain and opioid concerns often have complex psychiatric and medical histories. To provide the highest level of collaborative patient-centered care, conducting a thorough patient evaluation to determine the optimal treatment plan is a critical first step (Dansie & Turk, 2013). Using a biopsychosocial approach that incorporates all germane factors is imperative for maximizing the chances of successful treatment engagement and outcomes (Turk & Robinson, 2011). This approach includes attention not only to the information shared by the patient but also to other relevant data that may be helpful in decision making, such as assessment tools or screeners, notes from other providers when available, and details from prescription-drug monitoring programs. Real-world pressures and constraints, such as lack of time, can create barriers for the ideal comprehensive analysis, so it is critical at this point to acquire a full picture of the individual to ensure that important factors are not overlooked inadvertently. Missing nuanced details about family substance use or current mood lability can lead to adverse outcomes in the future.

https://doi.org/10.1037/0000209-005
Chronic Pain and Opioid Management: Strategies for Integrated Treatment,
by J. L. Murphy and S. Rafie

The evaluation often begins with brief education, explaining how a variety of factors shape the pain experience. Background on this complex process helps patients understand why psychosocial and other information is needed to determine the best next steps. Because similar messages often need to be presented numerous times before they are fully processed, key points should be introduced early and reinforced often. When possible, enlisting the assistance of other health care professionals, such as nurse care managers, may reduce the burden on a single provider; it also supports team-based care.

EXPLAINING THE BIOPSYCHOSOCIAL APPROACH

The biopsychosocial framework is the widely accepted approach for optimally understanding and treating chronic pain (Gatchel et al., 2007; U.S. Department of Health and Human Services, 2019b). Unlike previous pain conceptions that were purely or primarily biomedical, the biopsychosocial model understands the experience of pain as one that is multidimensional and formed by complex and dynamic interactions between patients' biological, psychological, and sociocultural factors (Engel, 1977; Gatchel et al., 2007). It takes into account the complex and interacting biological factors (e.g., anatomy, medications, hormones); psychological factors (e.g., trauma history, pain catastrophizing, learning, development); and social, cultural, and environmental factors (e.g., social support, ethnic identity, spirituality, poverty) that form the pain experience. It is important to stress that this model does not minimize the physical aspects of pain; rather, it provides an explanation for the ways in which various factors impact pain. Understanding pain as a complex experience helps individuals account for pain fluctuations and for variability between individuals with similar conditions. This model also supports the differences in opioid effects, given individual variance in how they are processed and used.

Clinical Conundrum: Meet "Jim" and Educate Him About Chronic Pain

Jim is a person with pain who reappears in this book through each phase of treatment; he is a fictional composite of many real cases. Jim is a 50-year-old man who presents with chronic low back pain that he manages primarily with opioids to "numb things a bit." He is married, works full-time in a physically demanding job, and describes himself as "barely getting by." He wants to reduce his opioid medication use because his doctor and family think he should, and he says he never planned to use opioids long-term. He discusses the challenges of waiting for medical treatments and describes being disappointed by the outcomes of procedures and medications.

The health care provider introduces Jim to the biopsychosocial approach to illuminate the dynamic nature of pain.

HEALTH CARE PROVIDER (HCP): I can see that the process of waiting for treatments can be frustrating, especially when you are unsure of what the results will be.

JIM (J): I am really tired of the runaround and just want to get some control over the pain. Right now I feel like my pill schedule is running my life. I'm hoping you have something different to offer.

HCP: Yes, the good news is there are many things that we can do. But first, I'd like to share some information with you about how pain works before getting into the treatment itself.

J: Okay, I'm listening.

HCP: As I'm sure you've noticed, pain is a very complicated problem. It is physical as well as emotional. You feel pain when your brain and your body communicate through your nerves. Those parts are responsible for creating every sensation you experience.

J: Like pain.

HCP: Right. So pain is processed and impacted by many things. It is affected by how well rested you are, your thoughts and stress level, and even your relationship dynamics and social experiences. So it is a physical sensation, but one that is integrated with a whole host of other things. That is why we call it the pain experience—it is about the whole person and all of the various factors that make up what is happening in this moment.

J: I have noticed that the pain feels worse when I'm irritated.

HCP: Perfect example. It's also a big part of why two people can have the same condition or diagnosis but describe the pain very differently. One may find that it is quite manageable, while the other feels like the pain is overwhelming. Biological factors are important, and we want to attend to them fully, but these other pieces make a big difference. Add in opioids, and it gets even more complicated.

J: That's why sometimes I don't know if the pills are even working.

HCP: It can get hard to piece it apart and figure out what's happening. Sometimes people get used to using opioids but find that they aren't helping much anymore. Fortunately, there are other strategies, which we will explore together, so you don't have to rely on a pill as your only option.

These conversations validate the patient's feelings and experiences and help to establish rapport between patient and provider. This may be the first time that the individual has heard about the complexity of pain from a health care provider. It is important for the provider to address concerns, unhelpful beliefs, or unrealistic expectations early and often. The conversation is an opportunity to learn about what is personally motivating and meaningful to the person with pain.

CLINICAL EVALUATION

A comprehensive biopsychosocial evaluation is the cornerstone for all treatment planning because the result will be used to determine the optimal approach to an integrated plan, which may include medication adjustments. Education about pain and opioids may be woven throughout as appropriate, but the aim is to gather relevant patient information across history and functional domains. People who need assistance with pain and opioid management are likely to have a variety of psychological symptoms, including depression, anxiety, mood swings, anger, irritability or decreased frustration tolerance, issues with concentration and attention, memory complaints, restlessness, and feelings of paranoia or panic. Psychosocial issues also frequently arise, including marital and relationship problems, absenteeism or poor performance at school or work, financial stress, social isolation, and loss of friendships. It is clinically useful to develop a structure of evaluating the whole person so that none of these important details are overlooked. This information will help the provider identify the optimal treatment pathways and determine how best to discuss those options. The language used when reviewing next steps directly affects the degree of openness and engagement. Practitioners must be thoughtful as they tailor the conversation appropriately and inquire about patient preferences.

Before beginning the patient evaluation, it is helpful for a practitioner to collect as many data points as possible to inform a sensible treatment plan. Several types of important information may be gathered. Output from a state-based prescription drug monitoring program (PDMP) provides facts about medications and medical providers. It is useful for the practitioner to see prescription refills for opioids and other controlled substances and to determine concurrent use of medications such as benzodiazepines. The PDMP also reveals any potential aberrant behaviors, such as obtaining similar prescriptions from multiple providers, which is key for risk mitigation. In addition, notes from previous health care visits can provide helpful background if they are available. They can clarify whether someone has consistently engaged in mental health care, physical therapy, or other recommended consultations. Records also provide insight into how the individual has taken medications over time, negative side effects, and longitudinal trends in pain intensity. Inpatient admissions for medical or psychiatric reasons, such as surgeries or acute instability, are useful, particularly if they involve an issue that the patient may be less likely to share, such as suicide attempts. Finally, providers can obtain various assessment tools to assist in evaluating pain-related functioning, attitudes related to pain, and opioid-related behaviors. Chapter 6 provides additional information regarding measurement options.

A thorough evaluation should assess the strengths and vulnerabilities of a patient by understanding their previous and current treatments, behaviors, and functioning. The clinician should focus on safety and function, risks and benefits. This focus requires consistent inquiries about what function "looks like" and how it is operationalized by the patient (e.g., a good day, bad day, typical day; treatment success or failure). Patient safety should be maximized. An overall goal is to better understand patients' relationships with pain and with opioid medications—how they think about them and what impact they have on daily functioning.

The most important information to gather during a clinical evaluation of a patient experiencing pain and managing opioids include the following:

- psychosocial basics, such as relationship status, children, occupation, residence, and religion or spirituality. These factors provide context and help the practitioner determine which ones may be of help or hindrance.

- pain location(s) or condition(s), intensity (e.g., average in last week), quality, and duration (i.e., number of months or years).

- functional impacts of pain in physical, emotional, social, sleep, occupational, and recreational domains. Asking about a typical day is often a comfortable way to inquire.

- current pain medication prescriptions. A practitioner may ask about how an individual uses medications (e.g., they may take less or more than prescribed) and then may consult PDMP information to confirm medications.

- all current and previous treatments for pain management, along with their effectiveness.

- current mood and related symptoms.

- previous and current psychiatric diagnoses and treatment, including hospitalizations. Hospitalizations are often related to suicide attempts, so this may be a fitting time for a clinician to broach the topic of self-harming behaviors.

- history of suicidal ideation and attempts, as well as current ideation, intent, means, and protective factors. Special care should be taken because individuals with chronic pain have an increased risk of suicidality (Petrosky et al., 2018; Tang & Crane, 2006) and prescription opioids introduce a means for overdose.

- current psychiatric medication prescriptions. Clinicians should consider concurrent use of benzodiazepines and opioids because of the increased risk of death from overdose associated with this combination.

- substance use, including details of previous and current use (e.g., type, amount, frequency, date of last use, context of use or relapse) and family history of substance use (i.e., a risk factor for opioid use).

Through the initial clinical interview, practitioners can identify individuals with additional mental health needs and refer for services as indicated. For example, someone who has a history of bipolar disorder who endorses labile mood and is not on appropriate psychotropic medication should be referred to a psychiatrist and stabilized prior to any changes in opioid analgesics. An individual who has a high level of anxiety and does not have adequate coping skills to manage mood symptoms should be referred to a psychologist for the development of cognitive behavioral skills either prior to or concurrently with opioid deprescribing.

Clinical Conundrum: Learning About Jim's Opioid Use

During the initial evaluation, Jim shares that he is not functioning well, is highly inactive outside of work, and is dissatisfied with his quality of life. The health care provider wants to learn more about Jim's relationship with pain and opioid medications and about their impact on his daily functioning.

HEALTH CARE PROVIDER (HCP):   When do you take your opioid medication?

JIM (J):   I take it when I wake up, when I'm leaving work, and before I go to bed.

HCP: Okay, so that medication is taken on a schedule. Do you sometimes take a pill as needed, or at other times?

J: Well, then I've got my short-acting ones that I take whenever I'm hurting.

HCP: Tell me more about how you feel and your thoughts during these times when you're hurting.

J: Sometimes it's the middle of the night, and I can't sleep because of the pain. Other times I'm just driving, and the pain starts up. Just last week, I got into it with my wife, and my back really started killing me. It's exhausting, and this is the only thing that seems to give me some relief.

HCP: I hear that—the pain is a constant source of frustration for you. Sounds like sometimes it's worse if you're stressed, or busy with physical activities, or it's just been a long day.

J: It just helps to release some of that, so I can just numb out and go to bed or relax.

HCP: I understand. The pills are for your pain, but your pain is also tied in with how you're feeling emotionally and physically. So, taking a pill can help you take the edge off, but it sounds like it's taking the edge off you generally.

J: Yeah, my wife would probably say so.

HCP: And you agree with her?

J: It's probably true. It's just the pain is too much; I need something to get through the day.

HCP: Once you take a pill, what happens after that?

J: If it's after work, I usually sit on the couch for most of the night. I'm worthless by then. I'm just wiped out after work.

HCP: Taking the pills isn't keeping you going so you can function outside of work. It's actually just your way of resting and recovering from the day. So it sounds like it's not helping you do more or interact better with your wife.

J: No. No, I come home and that's it. There's nothing left in me.

HCP: This vicious cycle you're in, we will continue to explore those patterns. Hopefully we can find some tools together for managing the pain and helping you feel less overwhelmed in general.

THE IMPORTANCE OF IDENTIFYING AND TREATING OPIOID USE DISORDER APPROPRIATELY

The majority of people who are prescribed opioids for pain do not develop problematic use or a substance use disorder (Cicero & Ellis, 2017). They may take opioids for a period of time and then taper off of the medications without difficulty, maintain manageable pain levels and functioning on low opioid doses, or take occasional as-needed opioids to assist with pain flares. Others, however, encounter struggles with opioid medications, even when they have taken them exactly as prescribed. This concept is particularly challenging—the notion that something prescribed by a physician for pain treatment could create dependency or even overreliance is challenging for many individuals with chronic pain. This challenge can make conversations around treatment more difficult (Sherman et al., 2018); patients are highly sensitized, and many are used to health care providers suggesting that they may be drug seeking (Buchman et al., 2016) even when their desires for medication feel necessary to address their pain concerns. They may have a hard time considering that the opioids they are using for pain control could be related to addiction: How can they be addicted if they do not get high and have never gone to the streets for drugs? People with pain often feel quite "different" from people with other substance use issues because they may have had a very different pathway to the present (Sherman et al., 2018). Prescribers may have their own feelings of guilt and responsibility, which add to the complex clinical interaction. The reality is that the line between opioid concerns and the presence of opioid use disorder (OUD) can be fuzzier than many providers would like. However, the persistent use of opioids leads to unintended consequences, such as OUD, for some individuals. The *Diagnostic and Statistical Manual of Mental Disorders* (5th ed.; *DSM-5*; American Psychiatric Association, 2013) definition of OUD is provided in Chapter 1, this volume; here, the focus is on what to do for those with OUD and the difficulties encountered in making these diagnoses.

A report from the National Academies of Sciences, Engineering, and Medicine (2018) states that "medications are irrefutably the most effective way to treat OUD—reducing the likelihood of overdose death by up to three-fold." Clinical practice guidelines agree that when the criteria for OUD are met, the evidence indicates that an immediate evaluation for medication-assisted treatment (MAT) is recommended (e.g., buprenorphine-naloxone, methadone, naltrexone; Bruneau et al., 2018; Kampman & Jarvis, 2015; U.S. Office of the Surgeon General, 2016; U.S. Department of Veterans

Affairs and Department of Defense, 2015). However, a U.S. Office of the Surgeon General (2018) study showed that only about one in four people with OUD (28.6%) received specialty treatment for illicit drug use over the course of a year. MAT, also referred to as medications for opioid use disorder (MOUD), relieves the withdrawal symptoms and psychological cravings and positively affects behavioral choices. These medications can be used safely for varying lengths of time, depending on patient need, and can be coupled with therapy to address other aspects of addiction. MAT is effective for reducing overdose deaths and improving retention in treatment as well as reducing illicit drug use. In addition, evidence suggests that medications such as buprenorphine-naloxone can be helpful for pain management, which is of concern when considering transition to MAT. The importance of identifying OUD and initiating MAT cannot be overstated. It is challenging to engage in treatment for chronic pain effectively if one's focus is on obtaining opioids. A person with severe depression ideally would be stabilized on antidepressant medication to maximally benefit from participation in therapy; this logic also holds for those with OUD. MAT should be employed so that individuals with chronic pain can engage and succeed in behavioral treatments.

While referral for substance use disorder evaluation and treatment is rarely an easy process due to stigma and other factors, individuals with chronic pain may display more resistance than those without pain. They may feel that they are different from people who abuse substances obtained illegally because, at least initially, they received opioids from a physician for a medical condition. In addition, people with OUD and chronic pain are often still experiencing high levels of pain intensity and pain-related impairment and may still feel that they need the medication to sustain their current level of pain management, even with the problems that opioids may have caused. Despite the many possible resistances and complications, MAT is paramount for treating OUD effectively, and additional time and sensitivity should be taken so that individuals understand its benefits.

Triage Options for OUD

The acquisition of information during the evaluation provides scaffolding for disposition decisions. When discussing treatment options for OUD with a patient, a practitioner must establish a warm and collaborative tone that prioritizes the needs and input of the patient. This is a time to discuss what the clinical picture looks like, based on the information obtained and provided. Sharing information about MAT in a nonjudgmental way and explaining how it can be helpful in transitioning away from the current patterns, including the ups and downs that are often experienced with opioid dependence, are encouraged. Patients should be informed that MAT is empirically supported as the best treatment for OUD and that it has helped thousands of others facing similar challenges. Presenting this information does not mean that the patient is ready to transition to an option such as buprenorphine-naloxone, but the provider has the responsibility to share their clinical recommendations, reassure the person, and provide information about safety and benefits. If the individual is open and interested, then ideally a warm handoff can be made to a provider who can assist immediately—delaying access to MAT can be the difference between life and death, positive engagement and continued dangerous behaviors (Kresina & Lubran, 2011). Often, individuals are not open to OUD treatment because they do not believe they have a problem or issue that requires treatment. Typical resistance to MAT and other recommended treatment options is discussed further in Chapter 5, along with ways to manage it.

Acknowledging Difficult Distinctions

One of the biggest clinical challenges for health care providers when working with individuals managing both pain and opioids is determining the difference between more commonplace issues that arise for individuals with chronic pain and potentially concerning opioid-related behaviors (i.e., those that warrant further evaluation and a shift in treatment approach). Both providers (Juurlink, 2017) and patients (Goesling et al., 2018) may have difficulty determining the harms and benefits of long-term opioid use, which can make these lines blurry. Patients may technically meet *DSM-5* criteria for OUD (American Psychiatric Association, 2013), but OUD is more difficult to identify when the patient perceives prescribed medications as helpful for pain, even in the absence of measurable gains. While this book cannot provide answers around such highly complex topics, it is important to acknowledge that many times practitioners do not know definitively how to categorize opioid use or behaviors, particularly in cases of multimorbidities. Examples of some of these tough questions include the following:

- Looking beyond the tolerance and withdrawal criteria, do you evaluate OUD differently in those who are prescribed opioids compared with those who are not?

- What should you do if a patient stops the taper plan when pain increases?

- Labels can be harmful sometimes; is it necessary to use the label OUD?

- How do you determine the type of treatment focus needed for each patient—do you center on pain, substance use disorder, or both?

- What if a patient with pain really doesn't want to reduce their opioids but is not misusing? Even if the benefit is unclear, is it okay for the person to stay on the meds?

Unfortunately, the answers to these complicated questions are scarce. Empirical guidance is lacking and often seem left to opinion—if you ask five different health care providers, you may get five different answers.

While much is still unknown, some things can be said with confidence. Evaluating each person carefully and formulating a collaborative, individualized and compassionate plan of care is foundational (U.S. Department of Health and Human Services, 2019a). The priority is to partner with patients and listen to their input with an eye toward prioritizing safety and minimizing risk. The most recent guidance from the U.S. Department of Health and Human Services (2019a) makes it clear that shared decision making is critical. The guidelines suggest that behavioral health support should be provided, that taper rates (when indicated) should be individualized, and that OUD should be evaluated as indicated and treated with MAT. But the HHS guidelines clearly state that "if the current opioid regimen does not put the patient at imminent risk, tapering does not need to occur immediately," and time should be taken to provide education and obtain patient buy-in to increase success of reduction. In such scenarios, tapers can be slow or paused as needed. For individuals with pain who also use opioids, integrated treatment options are scarce, but they are likely preferable for most people. While treatment programs that address both in the context of an ideal interdisciplinary setting are not available to most people, perhaps this area will see the growth needed to include many of the strategies set forth in this book. The OUD label can be helpful and even necessary in some settings to obtain access to MAT, although individuals may resist owning this diagnosis. Perhaps that is unimportant; rather, it is essential that people receive the care they need and that patients are not left to navigate their pain and opioids concerns without support. The strategies included in this book are intended to arm individuals with skills for managing and reducing such distress around pain and opioids.

Clinical Conundrum: Partnering for Success

Jim discloses the challenges he has faced because he has relied on medications as his sole pain management tool. The health care provider partners with Jim by using nonjudgmental listening, explaining without blaming, sharing impressions, conveying the safety and effectiveness of the plan, and reinforcing an integrated course of treatment.

HEALTH CARE PROVIDER (HCP): I understand that you received opioids from a doctor and that you have not taken them other than as prescribed. No one is suggesting that. I also understand from listening to you that the shift in how your medication will be prescribed has been frustrating. What are some of the struggles you've faced in using your opioid medication?

JIM (J): It has gotten to the point where I'm planning my whole day around when I take my meds. If I miss one or take it much later than usual, I feel even worse, so I have to try to plan ahead for where I'm going to be and how long I'll be gone. I almost have to think about it all the time because I don't want to end up in withdrawals.

HCP: It seems that you have developed a physical dependence on opioids. That is an expected part of the process, but it sounds like these medications have also become your main focus. From what you shared before, it's clear that they are not helping with pain management like they used to, although you've increased your dose several times. Plus, staying on top of when and how you use them is taking a lot of energy. That sounds pretty anxiety provoking and exhausting!

J: It totally is. But I don't know the alternative at this point. I feel stuck here.

HCP: The outcome of the evaluation will let us know what the best option for treatment might be. That may be to work together to reduce your opioids very slowly, in the structure of a well-rounded plan. For some, the best option is to switch to a different medication that helps minimize those ups and downs. No matter what, we want you to live more comfortably so that you can focus on things that matter to you.

J: I'm willing to give anything a try, but I'm also a bit afraid of what might happen if we start changing my medication. I wonder if I will be able to work.

HCP: Let's determine together what makes the most sense for next steps. I will see you again so that we can begin working on strategies to help with managing your chronic pain and medications. We will discuss some tools to put you in the driver's seat so you can go back to being in charge of your day.

CONCLUSION

The primary goals of the first visit are to complete the evaluation, understand the patient's perspective, offer psychoeducation, and establish rapport. There should be room for flexibility, since it is likely that the individual may need more time to consider options, reflect on their current circumstances and motivation, and determine the best starting point. Ideally, this conversation is collaborative, with both parties able to contribute and achieve a level of synchronicity for the future. There may not be complete agreement on what might be best; views on the best next steps may be inconsistent or even opposing. However, this first visit is the start of a trusting partnership for ongoing communication. It is also important to remember that this conversation may need to happen many times. Engagement in treatment is stepwise and evolves over time. Ideas about the need for comprehensive care are often new, and practitioners may need to repeat or present messages in different ways until they are eventually heard. Willingness to participate in treatments may take days, weeks, or months. It is important to answer all questions the patient has, not make assumptions, and be patient with the pace.

5

EXCHANGE EXPECTATIONS AND ADDRESS RESISTANCE

Following the completion of the initial psychosocial evaluation, the focus shifts to acclimating the patient to the process of engaging in collaborative self-managed care for pain and opioids. The plan is to provide a structured approach to psychoeducation, intervention, and monitoring treatment progress with an overall objective to build a set of tools for actively managing pain while reducing reliance on opioid analgesia. Ideally, this process empowers individuals to be informed and active managers of their own health care. The treatment focuses on learning strategies and skills to reduce the effects of pain and opioids on important life domains and goals, such as relationships, physical and mental health, career, spirituality, and pleasurable pastimes. The hope at this stage is that the patient understands behavioral approaches, such as those that are active and focused on fostering self-management, while the health care provider offers scaffolding for support and collaboration. The goal is to empower people to believe in their own abilities to respond to pain in a helpful way and not let chronic pain or opioids control each day.

https://doi.org/10.1037/0000209-006
Chronic Pain and Opioid Management: Strategies for Integrated Treatment,
by J. L. Murphy and S. Rafie

ESTABLISHING THE CONTEXT OF TREATMENT

Visits introduce new topics through psychoeducation, relevant skill practice, and goal setting for at-home practice. The health care provider should select treatment options based on what is most relevant for the individual. The content of these interactions will also include issues brought forth by the patient, such as challenges related to pain intensity and opioid use since the prior visit, broad health care issues related to their condition, and psychosocial stressors. The content that is covered in each appointment may need to be modified to address current significant or emergent issues. Because individuals in this population may be facing intense challenges with a limited internal skill base for management, it is important to attend to the possible topic du jour while returning to the focus of treatment. One way to do this is to connect the presenting concern with pain: Did the person notice how the situation affected their pain, thoughts, or opioid consumption? This connection can be a way to acknowledge what is being shared and to direct energy back to a purposeful discussion about pain and medication management.

The treatment is tied to the development of skills, such as graduated and paced behavioral activation, relaxation training, cognitive evaluation and reframing, pain flare-up and stress minimization and management, and pleasant activity scheduling. Skills are introduced with an opportunity to discuss how they might look in the person's life, and feedback is provided. For example, if it is appropriate at this visit to focus on flare-up management, the patient may share examples of behaviors that have created pain flares in the past. The provider would then discuss concrete ways that the patient can decrease the occurrence of pain flares (e.g., pacing activities) and determine a plan to address future flare-ups, as it is unrealistic to expect elimination.

All discussions should be collaborative and should incorporate the person's goals in the treatment strategy. Using strategies daily and gaining mastery and benefits through practice are emphasized. Patients should leave health care visits with concrete action plans for implementing these skills in their daily life and with and understanding of how the use of these skills will improve the management of pain and medications.

REALISTIC EXPECTATIONS

As discussed in Chapter 2, expectations are a powerful variable in pain outcomes (Fields, 2018). The discussions with patients should focus on realistic expectations for progress. Common amongst patients with pain is the belief that adherence to treatment recommendations should result in significant reduction in pain within 1 to 2 weeks. The expectation of rapid results, specifically regarding pain reduction, is not realistic and is unhelpful to the treatment process. While the person in pain is beginning to practice new strategies, they may feel more uncomfortable before improvements emerge. For example, the person may experience increased discomfort with behavioral activation and more movement. This discomfort does not indicate that damage is being done, but it is typically a side effect of a sedentary lifestyle and deconditioning. Providers should have a direct conversation with patients to help set appropriate outcome expectations with an ongoing focus on functional improvements, operationalizing what changes in a "pain score" would look like and mean in daily life.

Similarly, the treatment team should prepare the patient to expect that reduction in opioids may increase pain in the short term. Although the pain increase is temporary, the knowledge will help the person to set appropriate expectations prior to initiating the opioid taper as well as to moderate reactions once the taper has begun. The hope is that the person experiencing increased pain will have a more calm and normalizing response, instead of catastrophizing. An increase in anxiety about medication reductions should also be reviewed. Although anxiety mimics some withdrawal symptoms, the plan should not necessarily be adjusted. This normalization of experience should occur throughout the various phases of treatment. When deprescribing occurs, it is always sensible to review possible withdrawal symptoms and address concerns. This review is an important step because it allows the health care provider to share realistic expectations with individuals and to respond to questions, fears, or concerns that they have. Data illustrating the effects of opioid tapering can often be helpful in these conversations.

EVALUATING PROGRESS

The health care provider plays a vital role in reviewing the patient's beliefs about chronic pain management and the role of opioids. These discussions should happen early and often to provide adequate education to modify inaccurate or unhelpful beliefs regarding treatment and outcomes. The health care provider should impart information regarding typical outcomes (as noted in Chapter 2), measuring improvement, and identifying progress. The provider should specify that improvement is measured through function, reports on well-being, decreased pain interference in valued activities, and reduced reliance on analgesic medications. A big part of setting patients up for success is informing them that, with consistent use of skills, they will see progress within weeks; when using some tools, such as relaxation, they may see results immediately. Benefits come in a variety of forms and include increased energy, increased strength, improved mood, reduced pain-related fear, increased social participation, reduced anhedonia, and increased tolerance for physical activities. In the long term, many patients experience reduced frequency and intensity of pain flare-ups, improved sleep quality and quantity, reduced stress, and improved relationship functioning. The following case illustration shows how a provider might explain how progress will be tracked and what the patient can expect.

Clinical Conundrum: Setting the Stage

Jim has completed the evaluation, and he conveys his hope that this treatment will help eliminate his pain. The health care provider will offer psychoeducation, set realistic expectations, and review how progress will be evaluated.

HEALTH CARE PROVIDER (HCP):   We will work together in each meeting to develop skills and tools to help you live better with pain. My goal is to share what I know about dealing with the kind of persisting pain you have so that, moving forward, you can gain confidence in your ability to manage pain without relying on opioids or doctor's appointments as frequently.

JIM (J):   I'm hoping that I'll start seeing my pain is going away so I can cut back on these pills. Then I can start living my life again.

HCP: The treatment strategies that we will discuss have been studied for decades to see how well they work. We know that most people will function better and feel better using these approaches. That means getting more active in a safe way, feeling emotionally better, getting back to your life, and feeling more like yourself. The research says pain decreases a bit and quality of life improves a lot. For most people, just decreasing opioids does not change their pain much, but for some people, it actually improves their pain.

J: So it's not a fix, but will hopefully help with the pain some. Even if I just learn how to deal with it better, that would be a win for me.

HCP: That's a great way to think about it. Learning how to deal with it better by responding in ways that are to your advantage is key.

We will work on creating new habits to live your best and healthiest life every day.

J: That makes sense, and I am on board with that plan.

HCP: Great! So as we go along, we'll look for change in your mood, activities, use of medications, and the extent to which you return to important parts of your life, like family, friends, and hobbies. Of course, managing your pain better is an important goal for us, but we won't focus on your pain "score" per se. Because you have some pain most or all of the time, it's not the most helpful way to determine progress. Highlighting ways that your life is improving provides more meaningful feedback. Also, the changes in your medications may cause some fluctuations in how you feel until you have fully adjusted to a different dose. But reducing your meds slowly and thoughtfully, getting lots of input from you, should minimize that.

J: Okay.

HCP: So I will keep checking in about your mood, sleep, energy levels, and functioning in other areas that are important to you. I'll ask for updates about how things are going with your opioids and any impacts you may experience from changes. As you gradually test the waters with new activities and ways of thinking, you'll start to get some confidence back. Little by little, you should feel more confident and that you have more tools that opioids alone to feel better.

PREPARING FOR CHANGE

The overarching objective in treatment is to improve functioning and quality of life by increasing the use of wellness-focused self-management strategies for chronic pain and opioid management. However, learning to handle pain and opioid use effectively is a process that depends on individual awareness of what is currently unhelpful and how modifications may result in progress toward improved functioning and achievement of goals. Thus, while the clinical evaluation discussed in Chapter 4 will inform providers about appropriate treatment options, none of the options will likely work if the individual is not ready to change. Change is optimized by preparing individuals to adopt new behaviors and response patterns for pain and opioids, and this preparation includes exploring levels of resistance to change. This part of the process is critical because the population often enters clinical interactions with hesitation based on their experiences with the health care system, their conditions, and stigma within the social and political environment.

STAGES OF CHANGE

The stages of change were initially introduced by Prochaska and DiClemente (1982), who explained the process whereby individuals change problematic behaviors (DiClemente & Prochaska, 1982). The stages of change were initially introduced as part of their transtheoretical model to address alcohol use disorder (Miller, 1995). The stages focus on an individual's readiness for change, as follows:

1. *precontemplation*: the initial stage, during which the individual does not intend to change, may not realize the consequences of their current behavior, and is considered not ready for change

2. *contemplation*: the individual is considering how current behavior patterns may be problematic and believes there may be a benefit to change

3. *preparation*: the individual accepts that a change must occur and is taking steps to ready themselves

4. *action*: change occurs, including beginning new patterns, implementing replacement behaviors, and setting plans in motion

5. *maintenance*: continued progress toward the goal while monitoring for potential obstacles and overcoming as needed

Later iterations of the model also include a termination stage, in which change is sustained and permanently adopted. Relapse is a return to an earlier stage; during relapse, the individual learns to overcome barriers to sustained change. The stages in the model are relevant for all individuals making health behavior changes, including decreasing opioid use and increasing healthy lifestyle factors known to improve pain management. Research on populations with opioid dependence (Cavaiola et al., 2015) shows that most people going through medication-assisted treatment are in the precontemplation stage of change. This finding is a useful reminder that these individuals are often still considering whether they want to change.

Providers would benefit from taking a quick assessment of the person's stage of change so that they may approach treatment appropriately. The Pain Stages of Change Questionnaire, developed by Kerns et al. (1997), is a 30-item measure that can be used to identify a person's stage and to examine readiness to adopt a self-management approach to chronic pain. Using a 5-point Likert scale, individuals rate how much they agree "right now" with various statements about pain, such as "I have been thinking that the way I cope with pain my could improve" and "I have tried everything that people have recommended to manage my pain and nothing helps."

The process by which change occurs depends on where the individual lies on the stages-of-change continuum. The provider plays a significant role in advancing the patient from precontemplation to contemplation as the patient becomes aware of harmful patterns in their current pain coping. Individuals in pain may believe they have no alternatives to opioids and thus continue a steady regimen or increase their regimen of analgesic medications. Patients may believe the pain sensation that accompanies movement is harmful and thus remain inactive. As physical symptoms worsen and activity decreases, individuals' worsening mood often contributes to stagnation and increased reliance on opioids to cope. Providers must be sensitive to these beliefs and emotions as they address the knowledge gaps that lead to maladaptive behavioral patterns. Providing detailed education regarding the individual's condition and how to properly manage their symptoms is paramount in raising consciousness. With proper education, the foundation for self-management of chronic pain is set as people are motivated to adopt adaptive pain management skills. Furthermore, because many patients may be wedded to the belief that opioids are the only thing that can provide even minimal relief, it is sometimes a lengthy process to understand that there are other, more helpful ways to respond to pain (see Chapter 4, this volume, for more on patient education).

Although some individuals are unaware that a change is warranted, others want to make a change but are hesitant. Contemplators commonly worry about making a change to opioid medications they rely on, despite a desire to decrease or discontinue use. Contemplators may also fear they are unequipped to initiate activity without medical supervision or may doubt the effectiveness of proposed treatments. These questions and concerns create ambivalence about changing, which then negatively affects motivation and causes further delay in action.

MOTIVATIONAL INTERVIEWING

When assessing the individual's readiness for change, the provider may discover that the individual lacks motivation to change. Motivational interviewing (MI) is an empirically validated technique for helping patients increase their motivation (see Chapter 2). MI has become an increasingly popular strategy for increasing adherence to health care recommendations. Individuals managing complex pain and opioid regimens are often aware of the reasons to change their opioid use as well as the reasons to stay the same—there are pros and cons to both sides. As such, the provider's role is not to convince the patient to change but rather to serve as a guide in the process of settling the conflicts among their motivations, ultimately offering strategies and skills to aid the change process. Figure 5.1 illustrates the pros and cons involved in the decision-making process and reflects why ambivalence and relapse are so common.

The key components of MI are expressing empathy, identifying discrepancies between the current situation and hopes for the future, rolling with resistance, and supporting self-efficacy (Miller & Rollnick, 1991, 2002). As is common in many behavioral theories, the perception that the provider has empathy for the patient is central to establishing a trusting relationship between patient and provider. Identifying discrepancies between values and

FIGURE 5.1. Pros and Cons of Change and Maintaining

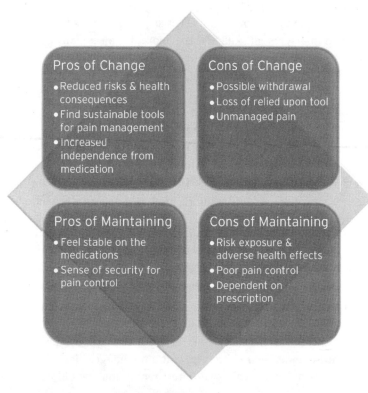

current behaviors allows the person to consider their goals and encourages making values-based choices moving forward. A point when the person gets stuck either in their progress or in their contemplation will always come. They may become frustrated or angry with the process. These emotions are not to be absorbed by the provider, and it is best not to engage in challenges or arguments, as these often lead to greater resistance (Markland et al., 2005). In fact, "rolling with" the person's feelings allows them to consider both sides of the issue and ultimately come to the conclusion on their own. Finally, the practitioner should reinforce the person's ability to overcome challenges and be successful with their goal. The practitioner's primary goal is to address and settle the patient's ambivalence so that they may progress toward readiness for change. These approaches help motivate patients toward adaptive health behaviors as their own change talk (i.e., the patient's statements indicating desire or reasons for change) often leads to choosing health.

One important tool for MI is a set of strategies known as OARS:

- *Open-ended questions:* questions that elicit lengthy responses, such as "How have your opioid medications interfered with your quality of life?"

- *Affirmations:* statements that express positive regard, particularly when appreciating a positive action, such as "You came to today's visit, despite your current pain flare-up, which shows your commitment to your goal."

- *Reflections:* rephrases or paraphrases of what the patient is communicating, such as "You're afraid you can't handle the pain with less medication."

- *Summaries:* statements that connect important themes the patient conveyed, such as

  "It seems your pain has been getting worse over time, despite the medications. Even though you want more pain control, it seems the medications aren't a real solution, especially considering the downsides to using them. You also mentioned you want to be healthier and more in control of how you feel each day. What would you like to do at this point?"

The provider must pay close attention to what is said and what is being conveyed during these conversations, being particularly vigilant to identify change talk. Specifically, the provider should listen for statements indicating the patient's reasons and need for change, their past experience with the change, and their desire to change. The provider should also listen for any statements regarding commitment, readiness, and steps taken thus far. Ultimately, the decision to change rests on patients themselves and is dependent on their values and goals. Regardless of patients' beliefs or choices, the provider meets patients where they are and aids in their change process.

Clinical Conundrum: Enhancing Motivation

Because of the clinical evaluation, the health care provider has learned that Jim experiences pain in his low back radiating to his right lower extremity. He has expressed uncertainty regarding etiology of his symptoms and a desire for medical intervention to fix the problem. He has completed numerous treatments with mixed results but no lasting benefits or changes. Jim is now on a steady dose of opioid medication, and he remains home when he is not at work. He is socially isolated and has few activities. The health care provider enhances Jim's motivation for change by setting the stage, raising awareness of the problem, becoming the guide, and reinforcing expected benefits.

HEALTH CARE PROVIDER (HCP):   I understand this has been a long and challenging process for you. Your life has changed in ways you never planned. You have worked with your medical doctors looking for a problem to fix, yet you are still with your pain. I know this has been frustrating for you. Are you open to learning about a different way to think about and manage your pain and opioid pills?

JIM (J):   Well, sure. That's what I've been asking for all this time, for a way to deal with this pain. I don't want to take these pills forever.

HCP: Since you have had pain for so long and tried various treatments, it is likely your pain will not go away entirely. This does not mean the opioids are your only option for dealing with pain, nor does it mean you have to keep avoiding the activities of life. How do you feel about trying out some new ways of dealing with this pain, to see if that might cut back on your need for as many pills?

J: I am open to trying it, but I have to say, I just don't see a way where I won't be totally useless by the end of the day.

HCP: Chronic pain does not respond to rest and medication the way short-term pain does. The science of pain management now shows that to properly address chronic pain, individuals must learn skills and tools to dampen pain signals and improve functioning. This lessens its negative impacts on your body and mind. We need to work together to understand your current circumstances better and to reconsider your limitations.

J: You know, I have concerns about the pain getting out of hand if we start messing with the medications.

HCP: As you are learning to deal with your pain independently, you will notice the intensity of your pain decreases some, and hopefully your reliance on opioids to deal with the pain will also decrease. That is one of our goals. You will form new ways of thinking, feeling, and responding to your pain.

ADDRESSING EMOTIONAL BARRIERS

Often patients with chronic pain who are using opioids have significant emotional barriers that go beyond a lack of motivation for treatment and change. It is challenging to contend with a health issue each day, and despite efforts to feel better, patients may understandably feel disheartened and disillusioned. It is important that a health care provider acknowledge the various negative emotional states that may be deeply interwoven with pain and opioid use and help patients work through these barriers.

Anger and Sadness

Adequate preparation for the biopsychosocial approach is one of the most important parts of treatment. This process is complex and includes addressing unresolved emotions, accepting pain as a condition, and committing to action. Depression and anxiety are typical emotional reactions to chronic pain, and anger is increasingly noted as a common experience that is important to address (Gatchel et al., 2007). Individuals often pass through stages of grief that include anger and depression before reaching acceptance (Kübler-Ross, 1973). Experiences of low mood and sadness for what has been lost should be validated and supported with empathic understanding. Health care professionals should support patients as they are processing thoughts and feelings regarding their pain and related life changes, until they are more at peace with the past and ready to move forward. The sooner patients can move toward acceptance that pain is chronic and can be actively managed and that life can still be meaningful, the sooner they can begin making necessary changes to improve functioning, including potential modification of opioid dose.

Hopelessness and Helplessness

For many months or years, individuals with chronic pain may have responded by avoiding physical and pleasurable activities, isolated themselves from others, and experienced significant changes in mood and general disposition

(Murphy et al., 2014). As people go through one unsuccessful treatment after another, they may feel as if the treatments were "failures," which is an unhelpful term. They will undoubtedly begin to feel hopeless and stuck in a seemingly futile cure-seeking cycle. Their feelings may present as resistance to biopsychosocial interventions. However, the patient is most likely not yet ready for change, and the health care provider should help to prepare them. If they have been using opioids for months or years, they may have become comfortable with this approach, despite undesirable effects such as sedation or social isolation. The health care professional should explore a patient's pessimism regarding changes, answer questions, discuss expectations for treatment, and suggest that they begin experimenting with therapeutic options to see if benefits occur.

It is also important to connect the dots between effective behavioral changes and reliance on opioids. If other paths to pain reduction are beneficial, providers can encourage individuals to explore them "as an experiment" to see the impact on function and need for medications. Repeated unsuccessful attempts to change should be reframed as learning opportunities rather than as failures. Without these discussions, patients tend to drop out of treatment because the expectations of patient and provider are misaligned (Prochaska & DiClemente, 1982). The health care professional must identify the individual's needs and start where they are—otherwise it is unrealistic to anticipate treatment success.

Clinical Conundrum: Addressing Hopelessness

Jim openly states that pain interferes with multiple areas of his life, and he feels that if he were pain free, his mood and family issues would resolve. He attempted an opioid reduction in the past, but he quickly returned to his original dose because he experienced increased pain and interference in work functioning. He is willing to consider reducing his dose again, but he is very fearful his pain and functioning will worsen. The health care provider shares information about the treatment, its scientific support, and instills hope.

JIM (J): Why would it work this time? I've gone down this road before. Once I was out of pills for the day, I was just left with no way to deal with the pain and felt awful.

HEALTH CARE PROVIDER (HCP): I understand your doubt and concerns. I can share that research tells us pain is informed by various factors, and we know that behavioral options are key to improving outcomes.

J: What does that mean, exactly?

HCP: Imaging of the brain shows us that by addressing how we think about pain, we can change the way we process pain and decrease its negative effects. We also know that certain behavioral techniques can improve how our bodies respond to pain so that it does not impact us in the same harmful ways.

J: Are we going to get rid of the pain somehow?

HCP: These types of approaches focus more on making decisions that allow us to gain control over it. These choices can dampen pain instead of amplifying it.

J: Okay, so the pain will still be there. That is still hard to accept. But it sounds like maybe I'll be able to deal with it better. I guess I'll give it a try; it couldn't hurt.

HCP: It is empowering to know that we have various options and strong evidence indicating that we can make the pain experience better. Now we have to be open to ways that we can take the reins and stop letting pain and opioids be in charge. This is not about coping better; it is about changing your relationship with pain.

Resistance and Ambivalence

Exploring resistance is a useful tool for more accurately gauging the person's understanding of chronic pain, the effects of chronic opioid use, and motivation for change. An individual may present as resistant in treatment for many reasons. One of the most common concerns that patients raise in an initial encounter with a behavioral health provider is uncertainty regarding whether the provider believes their pain is real. This concern demonstrates a fundamental lack of awareness regarding chronic pain management and provides an opportunity for the health care professional to offer education about the biopsychosocial model. Other patients may voice ambivalence regarding the active approach, which may be attributed to prior failed treatments, or they may doubt the effectiveness of the offered treatment. In these circumstances, the health care professional needs additional information to understand why the patient believes past treatments were not beneficial and what treatments they believe may be beneficial. Understanding a patient's reasoning provides insight useful for determining appropriate intervention and aligning with the patient.

To determine next steps, a health care professional must also assess the individual's beliefs regarding opioid analgesic use. Some may attribute their current level of functioning to their medication and may believe that they would be unable to function without it. Others may want to discontinue use of opioids, or even all medications, because of harmful side effects, but they may fear discontinuation from prior experience with withdrawal symptoms or lack of an alternative pain management plan. Another response may be total ambivalence regarding making any change to medications. The astute health care provider can draw from personal background, gleaned from the clinical interview, to identify areas for improved functioning and pain coping. The patient's values, including their reasons for pursuing this change, should be incorporated into this discussion. Furthermore, the health care provider should facilitate the patient's understanding of how opioids may be exacerbating their pain rather than decreasing it and should discuss how MAT may improve symptoms.

Health care providers should emphasize the need to build pain management skills, which can provide a bridge during the deprescribing process and beyond. The goal of exploring resistance is to increase the individual's understanding of their potential for self-management and reduced medication reliance. In the preparation stage, the clinician works with the individual in pain to enhance motivation for change and commitment to a plan. If they are convinced that opioids are the only things that work, it is not helpful to debate that point. Instead, a provider can suggest that although opioids have worked, other options have high quality evidence and may make opioid analgesics more effective and better able to promote functioning— approaching it not as "either–or" but as "and."

Clinical Conundrum: Addressing Resistance

Jim shares that he is maintained on 350 mg morphine equivalent dose (MED) per day. However, when a small reduction of opioid medications is mentioned as one aspect of a comprehensive treatment plan, he backpedals and says that he is doing well or at least well enough. He is upset at the suggestion to change his opioid dose. The health care provider revisits information shared, inquires about fears, gauges level of openness, and reinforces partnership.

HEALTH CARE PROVIDER (HCP):   The picture you just shared did not sound like doing "well" or even "well enough" since as you described it, your functioning and quality of life are poor. You told me that you have trouble getting out of bed, you are lethargic, and your mood is low. Is that an accurate reflection of what you described?

JIM (J): Well, yeah, but do you know how long I've been on those pills? And it was awful the last time I went down this road.

HCP: What fears do you have about making a change in your opioid dose?

J: That I'll feel physically sick, the pain, and if I'm not able to work.

HCP: Those are valid concerns. How do you feel the medication is currently helping your pain intensity or functioning?

J: It's not, really, but it keeps me going. I still feel awful most days, and I have zero energy.

HCP: Are you open to making a very small decrease in your opioid dose so that we can see the results and then follow closely to assess for changes?

J: I am open to the conversation because I want things to be better than they are right now.

HCP: We will make these changes slowly and together. Your feedback is important to me, and our shared goal is getting you back to where you want to be. We will practice lots of different techniques to give you more tools apart from the pills, all with the intent of having a better quality of life, where you can go to work and still have energy for other meaningful activities and interactions.

BUILDING SELF-EFFICACY

As individuals work through areas of resistance with the aid of the health care provider, they strengthen the foundation of understanding on which the process of change rests. When a patient develops increased awareness of problematic patterns and some insight into the need to make lifestyle changes, the seeds of self-management are planted. In the preparation phase, this awareness sprouts into confidence in and commitment to a change plan. The individual's expectations of themselves determines whether or not the new skills will be applied, to what extent, and with what level of perseverance in the face of challenges (Bandura, 1977). After the initial transition into the action phase has occurred, every behavioral decision will correlate with increased or decreased self-efficacy. Throughout each phase, the clinician should support the patient's growing sense of efficacy by highlighting willingness to face situations that are feared and were previously avoided.

Sample statements to boost a patient's sense of self-efficacy include the following:

- "You mentioned you felt more energetic after you walked daily for one week. That is evidence that by making a change to your actions, you can change how you feel!"

- "That's fantastic that you got through the flare-up using your tools and didn't increase your medications the way you've done in the past."

- "So you're noticing an improvement in your mood when you are making an effort to be more involved with your family. I know that has been challenging on some days, but it sounds as if the investment has been worth the payoff. I know they appreciate more time with you."

CONCLUSION

Reviewing expectations early facilitates patients' understanding of how progress is defined and helps patients shift from a pain focus toward a function focus. People who use opioid analgesic medications to manage their pain arrive to treatment with a wide range of attitudes about change. The stages of change can assist providers in identifying the degree to which patients are ready for change, from not considering any change at all to preparing to take action. Questionnaires can be useful in identifying a patient's stage of change, and providers can use MI techniques to help patients become ready to make changes. Regardless of where the person is on their journey, their considerations include positives and negatives of change and can come with a host of emotional barriers. Providers must recognize and address these ongoing issues, which tend to come up repeatedly as patients encounter obstacles or experience withdrawal symptoms or fluctuations in pain levels. Throughout treatment, emphasis should be placed on boosting the person's self-efficacy to promote independent and successful pain and opioid management. The careful consideration paid to readiness and resistances ensures that the patient is prepared to engage in treatment.

III

PHASE 2: ENGAGING IN STRATEGIES

There are no shortcuts to any place worth going.

—Beverly Sills

INTRODUCTION

This phase is where the work of behavior change begins in earnest. Preparation and exploration have now occurred, but those steps are academic until specific strategies for improving pain and opioid management are introduced and implemented. One of the biggest challenges for incorporating behavioral interventions is that they entail effort (Ory et al., 2010) and often require that individuals step away from familiar patterns. Patients are asked to participate fully in their treatment, which means not just attending meetings with health care providers but also practicing strategies in the hours when they are away from a clinic, office, or hospital. For many people, the suggested approaches may mean embracing a new and different perspective while allowing for increased discomfort to achieve improvements. For example, individuals with pain may be accustomed to using only opioids for anticipated or actual pain increases, but in this phase of treatment they will be encouraged to adopt different strategies, to minimize the presence of pain and flare-ups, and then manage them without relying solely on medications. The health care provider must be thoughtful in framing each intervention in a manner that is easily understood, supported by science, and seen by the person suffering as an avenue for an improved life.

Despite preparation, health care providers should expect fluctuations in patients' openness to the concepts and treatment interventions. These fluctuations are common for those struggling with pain-related suffering and their use of opioids. Individuals may start strong and be engaged and committed but express pessimism over time or simply miss appointments down the road. Some may vacillate week to week regarding buy-in because they doubt the effectiveness of behavioral tools or experience fluctuations in their willingness to participate fully. Reminders about the foundation for the strategies being implemented should be provided routinely and should address pain as a biopsychosocial and complex phenomenon for which no single approach or medication is sufficient. Furthermore, health care providers are encouraged to share the science to support self-managed behavioral approaches and the unhelpful nature of many automatic responses to chronic pain. Finally, individuals in this population may be sensitive because of previous experiences and may need to be reminded routinely that they are not being blamed for their pain or opioid use—instead, they are being empowered to learn new and self-managed ways to improve life, increase joy, and become more of who they want to be.

6 DEVELOP GOALS AND A TREATMENT PLAN

Engaging in treatment begins with collaboratively identifying personalized patient goals and determining the best clinical pathway to achieve them. Trust and rapport between provider and patient should continue to be fostered as a cornerstone for openness regarding motivational sources, current behaviors, and realistic plans for the future. Too often in clinical interactions, the nature of the problem and the course of treatment is dictated by the provider, with limited input from the patient regarding desires or direction (Institute of Medicine, 2011). This is a foundational error—setting up a treatment plan that follows provider objectives and is not highly informed by the person with pain is unlikely to lead to engagement in a process that is based on active efforts by the patient. It is imperative that provider and patient work together to determine the key issues and develop a plan for moving forward that is clinically appropriate, feasible, and patient centered (Epton et al., 2017).

https://doi.org/10.1037/0000209-007
Chronic Pain and Opioid Management: Strategies for Integrated Treatment,
by J. L. Murphy and S. Rafie

GOAL SETTING

A core set of cross-cutting general objectives for treatment serves as the base on which additional goals will be built. Every aspect of participation in treatment aims to (a) increase feelings of self-efficacy to manage pain and opioid use, (b) improve physical and emotional functioning, and (c) decrease pain- and opioid-related suffering. These objectives underlie the individualized and personally motivated goals that are developed with the patient.

Before delineating the best clinical course, health care providers must understand the desired outcome of treatment for the individual (Dunlay & Strand, 2016). A dialogue in which patients openly disclose their personal motivations for participating in treatment should occur—what does success look like for them? The provider helps patients first to identify what they want and then to develop a plan for how to get there. Research indicates that goals are a foundational part of change and that people are most likely to adhere to a behavioral plan if they have chosen their own goals (Epton et al., 2017). Goals serve several purposes: They remind the patient why they opted to engage in services and of the changes they would like to realize, and they provide practical guidance for how to move in the desired direction on a daily basis. Goals must be reassessed and adapted as needed to ensure that they are both realistic and inspiring, and often patients need a practitioner's help to develop a solid and feasible framework for attainment.

SMART GOALS

Although goal setting is often taken for granted, it is critical for positive patient experiences and outcomes. Many clinicians feel that they already "do goal-setting," but the process may be cursory because it lacks adequate time and reflection. Goal setting is the first step in developing a road map to an effective patient–provider pain management relationship. Goal setting communicates to patients that their input is necessary to guide treatment. Furthermore, it conveys that the intervention will be personalized based on their needs. This personalized care may be particularly important for individuals seeking improved pain and opioid management, as many people may feel that they have been subject to assumptions about their experiences. They may have felt disbelieved by the health care system or even unfairly labeled a drug seeker. Opening up a discussion about what the patient wants plants good seeds toward rapport building with a population that often does not feel adequately heard.

Breaking It Down

While there is no universally accepted approach to goal setting, several options are popular. Using a SMART goal structure is one popular choice— thoughtfully creating goals that are specific, measurable, achievable, relevant, and time-bound (i.e., SMART) provides a useful framework (Doran, 1981; Murphy et al., 2014). When developing a SMART goal, it is helpful to consider simple, specific questions. Table 6.1 provides sample questions and responses.

Breaking goals into smaller and more achievable parts can be helpful. For example, a patient indicates that she would like to begin quilting again. It is a pleasurable hobby that she gave up after pain and low energy became too overwhelming. The practitioner asks why she no longer engages in this activity, and she shares that her sewing table has an uncomfortable chair and is down in the basement. The last few times she used it, she ended up taking some opioids and going to bed afterward. Although her pain and sedation levels are relevant, a reasonable first step may be asking her husband to move the table upstairs to the office for easier accessibility. Another may be determining what form of seating may be more supportive and ergonomically appropriate given her pain limitations. What other steps should she take to accomplish the goal of setting up her quilting workspace? With this smaller goal she is not yet back to quilting, but it is a reasonable place to begin and establishes benchmarks that are achievable. Once this goal has been met, she can identify additional goals that help her to return

TABLE 6.1. Questions to Ask About a Goal

Ask	Answer	Answer	Answer
What?	Ride my bike	Use relaxation to reduce my PRN opioids	Visit my friend Susie
How often?	3 times per week	Daily or as needed	At least 1 time per week
Where?	At the park near school	In all settings	At her home 10 minutes away
When?	Tuesday, Thursday, Saturday	During pain flares and stressful situations	Wednesdays and Fridays are best for her
How much?	15-20 minutes	Use relaxation at least once before taking a pill	30-60 minutes

to her favorite pastime. She can consider engaging without concerns about dramatic pain flares or increased opioid use.

Breaking ideal goals into more manageable and less overwhelming parts can be particularly helpful when making changes to opioid medications. For example, if a patient's goal is to reduce opioid medication use by 50% in the long term, a feasible starting point may be to implement the use of relaxation before taking a PRN (i.e., as-needed opioid medication dose). This smaller goal may be the first step toward learning that a self-managed behavioral strategy can be effective in reducing opioid use. Continued success can breed confidence to speak with a physician about making a small change in dosing, something that may have been too frightening to consider previously. Each time a goal is realized, individuals are reinforced and experience positive emotions that can generalize to engagement in other areas.

Operationalize the Goal

One of the most common provider missteps is to fail to operationalize patient goals clearly. For example, consider an individual who states that he wants to be "more involved with my family." This goal is worthwhile, but without further clarification, there is no way to understand what that means or how the patient can achieve it. Follow-up questions are needed to create a clear roadmap to get there. Querying may reveal that he is most concerned with his fractured relationship with his wife, whose primary complaints revolve around his isolation at home and reluctance to join her when she leaves the house. The patient reveals that he misses his wife and wants to feel more connected with her, but he does not know how. Furthermore, he is afraid of disappointing her or, if he does engage more fully, of burdening her with his pain-related limitations or his opioid use. These feelings should first be normalized for the individual, as they are common for pain sufferers. The focus can then shift to a realistic initial step toward improving the distance from his spouse. Although the conversation started in the general realm (i.e., "I could spend more time around her at home"), with more discussion the goal became SMART: "Join my wife for at least 1 hour in the living room after dinner each night." After successfully achieving his goal and beginning to feel a renewed bond with his wife, he may set a new goal to join her for an outing during the week.

Generating Ideas

Another common challenge in goal-setting work is a dearth of ideas from the patient. At this point in treatment, individuals struggling with chronic pain and opioid issues have shared that they are not pleased with their quality of life; however, determining the areas of functioning that are of most concern or greatest import may require significant guidance from the provider. The provider should not make specific suggestions or inquiries; that is a common clinical pitfall. Instead, if an individual is struggling with spontaneous generation of goals, a provider can reference details shared in the evaluation: "Did you spend time discussing the stress you feel with your teenage son?" may be a reasonable query to determine if a goal about this relationship is important. Or perhaps a query may be focused on how to reduce unhelpful emotional reactions to a child, which lead to pain flares and opioid use. If the patient complained about decreased activity level due to sedation from medication use and concerns about increased pain, the provider can revisit that topic and ask what type of activation might be most meaningful to the individual. Once a direction is identified, using the SMART structure can help direct the conversation. Health care providers should be mindful of patient-centric care, even if it requires an extended investment of time initially so that clear goals can be established to guide treatment and increase motivation.

One Step at a Time

Clinicians often struggle with seemingly unrealistic goals from patients, which can be tricky. Having high aspirations is encouraged but should be balanced with what is achievable so that individuals are set up for success. How can both be achieved? The stepwise approach is often the best way to meet multiple needs. For example, a patient indicates that they would like to run a marathon, but their current level of physical impairment and functioning suggest that a marathon would not likely occur in the near future. Instead of discussing anticipated feelings of discomfort, a provider can ask what the first step to achieving this goal might be. If the patient is currently highly inactive, perhaps a gradual walking program to get them re-engaged physically makes sense as a beginning. Another approach is to follow up with questions about what running a marathon would mean to them or what value running served in their life. Insight into the essence of what made these activities meaningful might suggest other ways or modifications to achieve a similar experience.

Focus on Functionality

Discussion of the patient's goals may elicit unrealistic desires to be pain free or beliefs that significant reduction in pain will allow them to reduce their opioid use and return to their life activities. Perhaps the most challenging goal for providers is a pain level of zero. This goal may also be linked to opioid use: "If I were pain-free, I would not need to take opioids anymore." Some cases may be similar but less extreme, such as when the focus is to get to a pain level of 1 or 2 but the individual has had a relatively consistent pain intensity of 7 or 8 for the last 10 years. The best approach for this presentation harkens back to the core message: What is the functional goal? If this person's pain were a 2, what would that mean they could do? How would their life look different on a daily basis if pain were not calling the shots? The answers to these questions help the provider to understand how pain is affecting the person's life and what the person finds most meaningful. The goal is then translated for the individual instead of being about a pain score. If a person perceives that a certain pain intensity would allow them to be a better parent by participating in more activities with their child, for instance, then the SMART goal can be honed to reflect what that pain level means. Based on what the person is capable of today, for example, the SMART goal can be "to take my child to the park that is 10 minutes from our house at least once each week for 30 minutes." If a patient's goal is "to get off all pain meds," the approach might be similar. The provider should find out what that would mean to the patient—how would each day be different? Why are those things important? Taking medication reductions one step at a time, in a reasonable, paced way can also be built into a related goal. The discussion can help turn desires into a personal, actionable goal that is linked to function.

Clinical Conundrum: Developing Goals

Jim is having a difficult time identifying personally meaningful treatment goals even though he endorsed a high level of pain- and opioid-related negative interference. His only stated goal is that he wants "to do more." How is this lack of specificity best handled? The health care provider acknowledges his current state, operationalizes his stated goal, starts small, and determines first steps.

HEALTH CARE PROVIDER (HCP):   I know that pain and opioids interfere in your daily life. If you were able to do more without using more opioids, what would that look like for you?

JIM (J):   Do more of the things I'm asked to do, maybe actually go places when I'm invited.

HCP: How would a typical day be different?

J: I would pitch in around the house, and I would take care of the yard again. Especially the outside. It's all been neglected for so long.

HCP: More specifically, what is something you would want to do that you are not doing now?

J: Mow the lawn, pick up the dead leaves, prune some of the smaller bushes.

HCP: Got it. You want to take better care of your lawn and property but not use opioids to get you through it. Let's consider a first step that can help move you toward your goal. Of the things you mentioned— mowing, leaves, and bushes—which is most important?

J: I would say getting the bushes and hedges in shape. I used to be able to do it from the ground, but now it seems like too much reaching. Need to get a ladder or something. The last time I tried I was laid up for days and just tried to get numb from the pills.

HCP: As a first step, let's set a SMART goal for obtaining a small tripod ladder to help give you a wide, firm base so that you can benefit from the extra support and height. You may have to research it a bit and figure out which one is best for you, but it would be a step in the right direction. Does that sound reasonable?

J: I can do that. So, I don't have to start yet?

HCP: Let's make this as easy as we can by starting small. We can pick up from there after you accomplish that. Will you take this first step and then let me know how it goes?

J: Yes, I'll do that. I mean, that part is easy enough.

HCP: Great, it's a start! Once we have some motion toward what you want to achieve, the other pieces should feel easier.

DEVELOPING AN INTEGRATED TREATMENT PLAN

A treatment plan should be considered a living document that is revisited and evaluated on an ongoing basis. It sets a detailed framework for how to proceed clinically, providing guidance for both the health care provider and the person with pain. For the provider, a well-developed treatment plan assists with organization of current and future actions (e.g., consults) and provides a means for monitoring progress. For the patient, the plan can serve as a powerful motivating tool to delineate the purpose of treatment and a pathway to meet desired goals. Having a specified structure and focus for treatment assists with achieving favorable outcomes.

It is optimal to develop a pain and opioid management plan that is bio-psychosocial in nature—physiological, psychological, behavioral, social, and environmental aspects must all be considered. The patient's high-priority goals should serve as a guiding force in the plan, as everyone is unique with their own desires and needs. Patient and provider should consider how they will each contribute to the implementation of the treatment plan. The clinician makes needed referrals, but the individual will be doing the heavy lifting of implementing the plan, and the details of how that will happen are critical. When possible, the treatment plan should cut across health care providers and disciplines so that all members of the treatment team are on the same clinical course and working toward the same goals.

The plan is informed primarily by the individual's goals as well as the provider's professional input and expertise; therefore, the process of treatment planning should be fully collaborative. Parties work together to determine appropriate therapies that should be initiated. While there is no single correct format for a treatment plan, a typical plan includes the following components:

- basic personal information (e.g., demographics, social support)
- reason for treatment, diagnosis, treatment and medication history
- patient-centric treatment goals
- subjective and objective measurements of progress
- timeline for evaluation and reassessment

When determining where to begin, the provider should first consider goals and options for the treatment plan that are most accessible and build gradually from there. If someone has tried to decrease opioid use before and has been unsuccessful many times, the provider might begin by focusing elsewhere. For example, perhaps an individual uses opioids in part to increase distress tolerance of pain. Instead of focusing on opioids, the practitioner might implement techniques to help self-regulate physiological and emotional distress (e.g., relaxation) and to consider the role of unhelpful pain-related thoughts. Addressing these areas and practicing strategies successfully will likely make the next step of minimal changes in opioid dosage much more achievable. Anticipatory fear will be decreased as self-efficacy around managing challenging situations and emotions is enhanced. If someone is focused on physical goals to improve conditioning and decrease reliance on opioids for exercise, a referral to a physical therapist is appropriate and should help the person understand safe activity boundaries, limitations, and the recommended graded approach for achieving objectives. Discussion of pacing activities and behavioral strategies to help delay use of short-acting opioids can be incorporated in the earliest phases of treatment. Using the individual's personal priorities as the guide and establishing meaningful and achievable goals early on will help reinforce the benefits of self-management and staying engaged in treatment.

Whole-Person Planning

A comprehensive plan addresses the whole person. In addition to physician supervision and a clinician to help with behavioral strategies, the ideal approach may include a movement program (e.g., yoga, heated pool), peer support (e.g., meetings), recreational activities (e.g., cards, darts), or spiritual outings (e.g., church). Practitioners should use their clinical judgment as well as the patient's interests and individual goals to develop a meaningful and realistic plan. Unfortunately, many people have limited access to specialty care or other services. Some services may not be available in their geographic area (e.g., rural areas), some individuals may have financial restrictions, and some insurance payers may not support all appropriate care. Some individuals may prefer home-based, more convenient, or private options. It is important that health care providers think broadly and perhaps less traditionally when determining the details of the treatment plan.

Pharmacologic and nonpharmacologic options are part of most comprehensive treatment plans for pain, and additional considerations should be given to individuals who are also balancing opioid use or reduction. Numerous nonopioid pharmacologic agents can aid in pain management. While medications are always associated with indications and risks, recent data indicate that certain nonopioid analgesics (e.g., nonsteroidal anti-inflammatories, acetaminophen) may be equally or more helpful than opioids for optimizing pain-related function and have lower risk of adverse events (Krebs et al., 2018). In addition, adjuvant medications for pain (e.g., anticonvulsants for neuropathic pain, antidepressants) can offer benefits and may be underutilized. Other medical options may be appropriate as well and should be explored with the person's physician.

The treatment plan may also include technology for pain management, which can be accessed via smartphone, tablet, or computer. At the most accessible and basic level, mobile apps help to guide engagement in active practices such as relaxation techniques. Apps that focus on simply tracking pain, however, are far less helpful because they often draw attention to a pain number and encourage staying closely focused on sensory experience, instead of highlighting function and promoting self-management skills. A variety of good options for activity tracking have a price point that is reasonable for many people (e.g., pedometer, smartwatch). They provide some guidance on activity but mainly assist with increasing awareness of number of steps, heart rate engagement, and minutes of activity, which can be useful and motivating. These devices can also be used to monitor sleep. Virtual or augmented reality is also increasingly used for pain management and can be used to increase activity engagement or relaxation by providing an appealing immersive experience. Online platforms for home-based chronic pain management programs, and even more comprehensive functional restoration programs, are also increasing. Various podcasts or organizations provide support for individuals with pain (e.g., American Chronic Pain Association). Finally, for certain specialties that are in limited supply in some areas, individuals may be able to access health care providers directly through web-based care. Pain physicians and psychologists or addictionologists may be accessible with a computer or phone, Wi-Fi connection, and camera. These options provide ample opportunity for each individual struggling with pain and opioid issues to develop a care plan that includes the services that they want and need, using a variety of treatment delivery routes.

Differing Opinions: When Patient and Provider Disagree on the Plan

For individuals who have been prescribed opioids, the guiding force in planning should be to carefully weigh the risks and benefits of use. When someone is interested in or open to reducing opioids and that is the clinical recommendation, the conversation is typically straightforward and without significant strain. However, opioid reduction is often indicated for individuals who object to decreasing most vehemently—people who need assistance the most may want it the least. It is generally agreed that if opioids have no functional benefit, reduction should be discussed, as is the case with any medication. If a reasonable trial has occurred and a medication is not helping, it is not sensible to continue. However, the opinion of the patient may differ from that of the health care provider or family. The individual with pain may insist, despite the evidence, that the opioids are helping, even when others see decline and lack of benefit. Especially in high-risk situations (e.g., daily dose is escalated, history of substance use, untreated obstructive sleep apnea), prescribers justifiably feel that an opioid regimen should not continue solely based on patient preference. As discussed in Chapter 4, these clinical scenarios pose the most challenges for all parties because of the lack of synergy regarding what the treatment plan should be. Health care providers can help facilitate a conversation that leads to collaboration and agreement across the group by using the following strategies in interactions related to opioid tapering:

- *explore and listen:* Allow individuals to share their concerns about opioid reduction. "What would a change mean for you?"

- *reassure and validate:* Provide empathy and reassure that you will not abandon them. "I want your input and understand your concerns."

- *educate and reframe:* Share information about opioids and what is known about the effects of reduction. "We know that opioids bring risks we want to avoid, and they may actually be increasing your sensitivity to pain. We want to find a combination of treatment options that will change your experience with pain for the better."

- *partner and start small:* Confirm that you will evaluate regularly, make changes as indicated, and encourage a slow and comfortable tapering pace. "We are in this together and are not in a hurry."

Clinical Conundrum: Discussing Medication Goals

Jim is joined by his wife and expresses hesitation about making changes to his opioid dose. While he is unsure it is providing much help at this point, he is also concerned that a reduction may lead to more pain and problems than he is already experiencing. His wife shares that she feels she has "lost him" because of his level of sedation and social isolation. Despite her feelings and the clinical recommendations, he remains hesitant. How is this best handled? The health care provider encourages taking the first step, starting small and reassessing often, being prepared for challenges, and easing the transition.

HEALTH CARE PROVIDER (HCP):   You have been taking opioids for many years, and it is understandable that the thought of a change is scary. Starting is the hardest part for most people, but if you are willing to give it a go, things get easier after this.

JIM (J):   It was just such a disaster the last time. I wasn't able to go to work, I felt awful, and I mostly laid in bed until my doctor changed my prescription back. I really don't want to go down the road of these big changes again.

HCP: Let's make the smallest change possible, how does that sound? You can let me know how it goes, and we will take it from there. You are in control, and we will work together closely the whole way.

J: How small are we talking here? Am I going to feel it?

HCP: With a slow and thoughtful reduction made with your input, the negative effects should be minimized. It is possible that your pain may increase slightly, but this is not the pain you have to live with forever, and this does not mean that your chronic pain is getting worse. It is also possible you may not notice any significant changes. There is variability across individuals, which is why I will check in with you regularly.

J: That was the worst part. I was going through it alone at home without anyone really even asking how it was going. I've been on those pills for so long now that coming off of them is going to be rough, I know it. It would help if I had someone checking in.

HCP: Absolutely! Collaboration is part of making this a successful process for you. And in the meantime, it will be helpful for you to learn about other strategies that can help you manage your pain and improve the opioid tapering process. Let's make sure you are using what we know works. We will work toward your goals of getting more quality time with your wife, pitching in around the house, and taking care of your yard. It's a process that we will work through one step at a time.

MEASUREMENT

While not required, using measures early in treatment to help establish a baseline and inform possible goals and treatment choices is strongly recommended. Assessment throughout the treatment process offers many pragmatic benefits. Clinically, it provides additional data when the patient presents, and it indicates growth or lack of improvement throughout treatment. Assessment information is used to select clinical interventions, troubleshoot current barriers, and guide next steps. Furthermore, the data provide evidence indicating whether the intervention is effective for the patient; this information can be used directly in clinical care to reinforce patients' progress and successes. Data can also inform the ongoing use of behavioral medicine strategies for individuals with pain by elucidating added value to patients themselves as well as to other providers. In addition, measurement can help guide the intensity of treatment and involvement of individuals from other disciplines and consultations. For example, someone with high levels of pain catastrophizing may require referral to a pain psychologist who can focus on how to affect mindset regarding pain and opioids before a deprescribing effort can commence. Basic information about some of the most useful constructs is provided in Table 6.2; the table also includes tools to assess pain and opioid use, with a focus on measures that are most clinically useful. Please note that this list is not meant to be comprehensive or exhaustive. Resources such as the Initiative on Methods, Measurement, and Pain Assessment in Clinical Trials recommendations (IMMPACT; Dworkin et al., 2005) and more recently Kroenke (2018) offer helpful insights on measurement considerations in research and practice.

TABLE 6.2. Tools for Measuring

Focus of measurement	Tool	Description
Pain intensity	Pain Numeric Rating Scale (NRS; Jensen et al., 1986)	11-point scale from 0 (*no pain*) to 10 (*worst pain imaginable*). It is used across health care systems and settings and has been validated as a treatment outcome measure (Dworkin et al., 2008; Jensen & Karoly, 2001).
Pain-related functioning or interference	West Haven–Yale Multidimensional Pain Inventory (WHYMPI; Kerns et al., 1985)	52-item assessment measured on a 7-point Likert scale; well-validated measure of several important dimensions of the chronic pain experience. It is divided into three parts and includes domains such as pain's perceived interference in areas such as vocation and life control, role of spouse or significant other, and engagement in everyday activities.
	Pain Outcomes Questionnaire-Veterans (POQ-VA; Clark et al., 2003)	45-item, multidomain instrument developed and validated specifically for veterans. Scales include pain-related interference with negative affect, mobility, vitality (i.e., strength and endurance), and pain-related fear (i.e., avoidance motivated by fear of pain, injury, or reinjury). Versions are available for different treatment statuses (e.g., initiation, discharge, follow-up).

(continues)

TABLE 6.2. *(Continued)*

Focus of measurement	Tool	Description
	Brief Pain Inventory–Long Form (BPI; Cleeland & Ryan, 1994)	32-item inventory that assesses the severity of pain and its impact on functioning; assesses additional information that may be clinically useful, such as pain quality. The IMMPACT panel recommends the interference items of the BPI for assessment of pain-related functional impairment (Dworkin et al., 2005).
Pain intensity and functioning or interference (brief measures)	Brief Pain Inventory–Short Form (BPI; Cleeland & Ryan, 1994)	15 items focused on self-report of presence, location, and intensity of pain, followed by treatments used and relief gained. The last seven items are recommended by IMMPACT for assessment of pain-related functional impairment (Dworkin et al., 2005). The short-form BPI is used widely and much more often than the long form; it is available in numerous languages.
	PEG (Krebs et al., 2009)	Ultra-brief measure derived from the BPI; three items that assess average pain intensity (P), pain's interference with enjoyment of life (E), and its interference with general activity (G). The PEG is often used in settings such as primary care because it is straightforward and practical.
Pain readiness to change	Multidimensional Pain Readiness to Change Questionnaire–2 (MPRCQ2; Nielson et al., 2003, 2008, 2009; brief version, Nielson et al., 2009)	69 items in two sections, with nine subscales (i.e., exercise, task persistence, relaxation, cognitive control, pacing, avoiding pain contingent rest, avoiding asking for assistance, assertive communication, use of proper body mechanics); measures readiness to adopt various pain management and coping strategies.

TABLE 6.2. *(Continued)*

Focus of measurement	Tool	Description
	Pain Stages of Change Questionnaire (Kerns et al., 1997)	30-item measure used to evaluate readiness to adopt a self-management approach to pain management using established stages of change.
Pain catastrophizing	Pain Catastrophizing Scale (PCS; Sullivan et al., 1995)	13-item self-report measure of the tendency to ruminate, magnify, or feel hopeless (i.e., catastrophize) about pain. Each item is rated on a scale from 0 (*not at all*) to 4 (*all the time*), with a total summed scale score ranging from 0 to 52. A score of 30 or above is suggestive of clinically relevant levels of catastrophizing.
Self-efficacy	Pain Self-Efficacy Questionnaire (PSEQ; Nicholas, 1989, 2007)	10-item measure to assess confidence in ability to do tasks and activities despite pain. Scores can range from 0 to 60, with higher scores indicating greater self-efficacy for managing pain. A two-item version is also available.
Opioid use	Prescription Drug Use Questionnaire–Patient Version (PDUQ-p; Compton et al., 2008)	31-item questionnaire designed for self-administration by patients with chronic nonmalignant pain who are also on opioid therapy. Derived from the original clinician-administered tool.
	Prescription Opioid Difficulties Scale (PODS; Banta-Green et al., 2010)	Assesses problems and concerns related to opioid use from the patient's perspective. One eight-item subscale assesses psychosocial problems attributed to opioids (e.g., loss of interest in usual activities, trouble concentrating); another eight-item subscale assesses patients' opioid control concerns (e.g., preoccupation with use of opioids, inability to control use).

(continues)

TABLE 6.2. *(Continued)*

Focus of measurement	Tool	Description
	Current Opioid Misuse Measure (COMM; Butler et al., 2007)	17-item self-assessment measure using a 5-point Likert scale to identify individuals with chronic pain who are taking opioids and have indicators of current aberrant drug-related behaviors. Questions encapsulate signs and symptoms of drug misuse, emotional and psychiatric issues, evidence of lying, doctor visitation patterns, and medication noncompliance.
Mood	Profile of Mood States (POMS; McNair et al., 1971)	65 self-report items rated on a 5-point Likert scale. It is used to assess transient, distinct moods. IMMPACT recommends POMS for measuring emotional functioning in chronic pain trials (Dworkin et al., 2005).
	Patient Health Questionnaire–9 (PHQ-9; Kroenke et al., 2002)	Nine-item self-report measure of depressive symptom severity. Scores range from 0 to 27, with higher scores indicating greater severity. PHQ is a well-validated, widely used measure.
	Beck Depression Inventory–Version II (BDI-II; Beck et al., 1996)	21-item self-report measure of depression symptoms, with each item scored on a 0–3 scale. Severity is reflected in a total score reflecting minimal (range 0–13), mild (range 14–19), moderate (range 20–28), or severe depression (range 29–63).
	Generalized Anxiety Disorder–7 (GAD-7; Spitzer et al., 2006)	Seven-item index of anxiety symptom severity with high reliability and validity. Scores range from 0 to 21, with higher scores indicating more severe anxiety.
	Beck Anxiety Inventory (BAI; Beck et al., 1988)	21-item questionnaire assessing the intensity of anxiety symptoms in the past week. Total scores range from 0 to 63, with higher scores indicating more severe anxiety symptoms.

TABLE 6.2. *(Continued)*

Focus of measurement	Tool	Description
	Patient Health Questionnaire-15 (PHQ-15; Kroenke et al., 2002)	15-item measure assessing somatic symptom severity. Cutoff points of 5, 10, and 15 represent mild, moderate, and severe symptom levels.
Sleep	Insomnia Severity Index (ISI; Morin et al., 2011)	Seven-item self-report questionnaire assessing the nature, severity, and impact of insomnia, measured on a 5-point Likert scale. A total score indicates the absence of insomnia (0-7), subthreshold insomnia (8-14), moderate insomnia (15-21), or severe insomnia (22-28).
	Pittsburgh Sleep Quality Index (PSQI; Buysse et al., 1989)	19-item self-rated questionnaire evaluating subjective sleep quality over the previous month, with seven clinically derived component scores, weighted equally from 0 to 3. The component scores are added to obtain a global score ranging from 0 to 21, with higher scores indicating poor quality sleep.
Multiple factors	Patient Reported Outcome Measurement Information System (PROMIS) pain-related measures (Cook et al., 2016)	Set of measures created by the National Institutes of Health and used across studies and clinical populations. The pain domains include item banks for pain interference and pain behavior and measures of pain intensity and quality (Revicki et al., 2009). IMMPACT recommends the core measures for pain clinical trials (Dworkin et al., 2005).

IMMPACT = Initiative on Methods, Measurement, and Pain Assessment in Clinical Trials.

CONCLUSION

Collaboration is the key for setting meaningful goals and establishing a realistic treatment plan. Health care providers help individuals uncover the will or motivation toward a goal and work collaboratively on the way to get there. It is critical to help patients communicate openly and honestly about their motivations for treatment and their desired outcomes. Often, individuals feel overwhelmed and helpless in the face of previous unsuccessful attempts to minimize pain or reduce opioids; therefore, both exercising patience and focusing on achievable steps to improve confidence and self-efficacy are needed. At this point in treatment, the focus should be on operationalizing goals so that a clear pathway for progress is set. With each success, a reevaluation of updated objectives or changes to the treatment plan may need to occur. Particularly when considering medication changes, it is important to support patients and guide them in understanding how they might best achieve their goals; such guidance may include recommendations for additional treatment. The addition of measurement can shed much-needed light in the most complicated situations and may clarify considerations for the treatment plan and areas of emphasis. By thoughtfully developing specific goals and a patient-centered treatment plan, a practitioner sets the path for acceptance of effective strategies for managing pain and opioids.

7 PRACTICE HELPFUL STRATEGIES

Many effective behavioral strategies can be employed to assist those who have chronic pain and also want to minimize their use of opioid medications. The following components in this chapter illustrate the core integrated interventions for clinical work with this population. Of explicit note, reducing opioid use should be approached under medical supervision and with careful planning. At times, patients may have a medical need to decrease opioids urgently, especially if they are in serious danger resulting from medical complications, overdose, or other highly risky behaviors (Fenton et al., 2019). Some with opioid use disorder (OUD) may have transitioned to another medication and stabilized. In any of these cases, the use of an effective pain medicine will help decrease distress related to pain and opioids. The strategies will promote active management and assist in minimizing the fluctuations in both pain and opioid use that are a primary struggle for the population (Henry et al., 2019).

https://doi.org/10.1037/0000209-008
Chronic Pain and Opioid Management: Strategies for Integrated Treatment,
by J. L. Murphy and S. Rafie

RETHINK IT

The role of thoughts in all aspects of human experience is central. Thoughts mediate how individuals process and respond to events in their internal and external environments. What people say to themselves can either facilitate or hinder positive outcomes of treatment and in life in general (Beck et al., 1979; Tota-Faucette et al., 1993). Unfortunately, since pain is a persistent unpleasant stimulus, it sets the stage for an increase in thoughts that amplify the pain experience (Sullivan et al., 2001). Sometimes patients find it hard to pay attention to anything but pain. If pain fails to improve over time, individuals' thoughts may become increasingly pessimistic and may exert a negative force in the pain experience. "Stinking thinking," as it is sometimes referred to in substance use settings, is ubiquitous, but these thoughts are often automatic and outside of conscious awareness (Beck, 2005; Ellis & Velten, 1992). Despite that, they have the power to dramatically shape emotions and actions (Beck, 1964). For that reason, recognizing and managing unhelpful thoughts is a cornerstone to effective behavioral management of pain and opioid use. In particular, pain-related catastrophizing thoughts have been identified as a potent psychological factor. The tendency to catastrophize plays a key role in pain-related functioning, mood, treatment outcomes, and disability status (Crombez et al., 1999; Sullivan et al., 2001). In addition, imaging indicates that the brain changes as a result of catastrophizing—the more that people catastrophize, the more pain-related areas of the brain are activated (Beck, 2008; Chehadi et al., 2017; Hubbard et al., 2014; Jensen et al., 2015). They may have heard feedback in health care settings suggesting that they are a "drug seeker" when they have presented with a desperate desire for pain relief. They may have struggled to justify their opioid use, even when it has been low dose and as prescribed. Before beginning a therapeutic relationship, they may feel or be defensive because previous experiences made them less open to a discussion about the role of thoughts.

At the outset of any discussion regarding the role of thoughts, it is best to help patients connect with their own experiences. Instead of starting with a lecture about the ways in which certain thoughts may generate unwanted consequences, a provider can help patients recognize the impact of thoughts in their own words, which is central to understanding their power. One strategy is to elicit personal examples so that people can organically examine their experiences; this is the route to insight and motivation for change. For most individuals, daily life is rife with examples in which unhelpful thoughts prevail (e.g., traffic, lines). The patient may have many accessible examples from the clinical interaction thus far that are linked to thoughts that did not improve the moment or mood. In addition, it may be helpful for the provider to use a metaphor or analogy to illustrate the power of thoughts, attention, and attribution. For example, for reasons of survival, humans are programmed to attend to stimuli that may be life-threatening or at least harmful. Things that are fear-relevant, such as snakes or spiders, are recognized more quickly than stimuli such as flowers or butterflies, and they demand more attention and emotion. This attentional load is part of why chronic pain is so challenging—although persistent pain does not indicate that life or limbs are acutely threatened, it demands the same level of attention as it would in the case of acute pain and imminent danger. Spending time increasing awareness of chronic pain-related thoughts can be particularly useful in combating their negative impacts.

Through an interactive conversation, health care providers should clarify that the discussion is about how perception of pain plays a key role in dampening or amplifying the experience. The message is not that the person is at fault or that the person should "just think differently and you won't have pain." Rather, it is an acknowledgment of the biopsychosocial model—various factors impact pain, for better and for worse. Some parts of the pain experience cannot be altered (e.g., history of a torn ligament), but fortunately others, such as thoughts, are highly malleable. It is about the meaning that we give pain and allow it to have. Increasing the use of tools to manage cognitive responses to pain and take control of the pain experience should be emphasized as an empowering part of the treatment process.

Focusing on changing unhelpful thoughts should not be characterized as a means to "cope better"—science provides perhaps the most convincing evidence that thoughts and expectations impact the pain experience and the effects of opioid medications. In one powerful study (Wager et al., 2004), a research team placed participants in functional magnetic resonance imaging (fMRI) scanners and induced pain via a heat stimulus, which was rated in the moderate range on average, equivalent of a 6.6 on a scale from 0 (*no pain*) to 10 (*worst pain imaginable*). All participants received a potent opioid through an IV line. Although the opioid dosing never changed, participants reported pain of 3.9 after they were told the medication was delivered; when they were told the medication was stopped, they reported pain of 6.4 (almost the same as prior to any analgesic). Importantly, the medication dose never varied, but the fMRI suggested that beliefs related to the opioid led to changes in the brain and blood flow. In other words, individuals experienced less pain if they expected that they would, even in the absence of any treatment changes. This finding can and should be shared with patients, as it clearly demonstrates the role of thinking and expectations in the pain and opioid experience. Many other studies support the role of thinking in the outcomes of pain treatment, including surgery, hospital stays, and pain chronicity; research indicates that thoughts are directly associated with pain perception (Lawrence et al., 2011; Seminowicz & Davis, 2006; Seminowicz et al., 2013; Shpaner et al., 2014).

Automatic but Changeable

Since many thoughts occur outside of conscious awareness, they may affect pain in ways that are difficult to discern. Identifying thoughts is often far more challenging than identifying feelings. Experiencing frustration or sadness is easier to label than the thoughts that precede or accompany them. However difficult, health care providers should use examples to connect feelings with the perceptions that surround them, demonstrating the role of both feelings and perceptions in the processing pain and daily life.

Examples of unhelpful thoughts that capture distress around pain and opioids are included in Table 7.1. After thoughts that may amplify unhelpful aspects of experience are identified, the next step is considering how to rethink them in a more balanced way. Instead of focusing on the veracity of a cognition, the patient should evaluate whether the thought serves them—does it build them up or bring them down? Does it lead them down a dark path or into a more neutral or lighted one? Providers can examine and evaluate these ideas with this approach in mind. Many available resources provide helpful tools for reframing thoughts.

TABLE 7.1. Rethinking Unhelpful Thoughts

Unhelpful thinking	Rethinking
That's it; I can't take this pain. I need to double my dose of meds just to get through this.	This is challenging, but before I take opioids I am going to try and see if the relaxation helps.
I can be happy with life only if I am pain free. I feel so useless. Even though my meds make me feel groggy and out of touch with my family, it's better than pain.	I get that my pain may never be a zero, which is hard to accept sometimes. Despite that, there is a lot I can do to live a full life. I don't want to just sit at home and feel out of it all day. I want to start living again.
I knew that this new medication wasn't going to be enough for my pain. These doctors are always wrong. They don't know what I go through, and I wonder if they even care.	The reality is that the opioids only helped my pain a little and they made me feel like a different person. Even though I feel alone sometimes, I know the team is trying to help me. I'll keep working with them and do what I can to get my pain under control.

Clinical Conundrum: Cognitive Reframing

Jim arrives to a follow-up visit after a sleepless night, struggling with his pain, and expresses helplessness regarding self-managing his pain. The health care provider takes this opportunity to discuss the role of our thoughts in experiencing pain, and together they practice rethinking, or reframing, his unhelpful thoughts.

HEALTH CARE PROVIDER (HCP):   Last night was a particularly rough night. I imagine today felt long.

JIM (J):   I was dozing off during my break at work and couldn't wait to leave. I feel like I'm losing, and the pain is winning. It's so frustrating. It seems like anything would be better than being in pain all the time. I'm tired of feeling useless.

HCP: You are more down today than I've seen you. It sounds like you are having a lot of dark thoughts about your pain

J: Well, you're seeing me on one of my bad days.

HCP: Not sleeping much last night is clearly affecting you. Sometimes when we are more stressed or down, the tone of our thoughts changes, too. Sometimes our brains come up with untrue thoughts, or just unhelpful thoughts, when we're feeling poorly. These unhelpful thoughts can amplify pain, making it feel worse and harder to deal with. Have you noticed these thoughts breeding more of the same? Getting caught in a downward spiral?

J: Oh, yeah, it just goes on all night. Then I feel my neck and shoulders tensing up, and sleep gets further and further away.

HCP: So, you know how our thoughts can cause us to feel worse and affect what we do. Would you be open to talking through some of the thoughts you've expressed today?

J: Sure, we can do that. I know I'm down on myself today. I can feel it.

HCP: There is a chance we can use the power of your thoughts to help you rather than to get you more down. You said anything is better than being in pain all the time and that you feel useless. Tell me more.

J: It's just how I feel. It is too much.

HCP: When you have these thoughts, how do they make you feel? We know that feeling and thinking are two different things but are closely connected. Are those thoughts I mentioned serving a helpful purpose for you?

J: No, they aren't helpful. They are the opposite of that. But I don't know how to stop them. I get really down.

HCP: So they make you feel more sad and depressed. I understand and want to see what we can do to lessen this type of thinking. It opens up the gate for more pain and more distress to walk right in. And we can say, for example, that feeling useless is not the same as being useless, wouldn't you agree?

J: Right, yeah. I guess I see where you're going. I know it doesn't help. And I know I'm not totally useless, of course.

HCP: Okay, then, how might you rethink what you said?

J: It's not as bad as I sometimes say and think it is. I am still working and providing for my family. Those parts are good. The pain is really bad, but at least I'm figuring out some ways I can get through it, and that helps me mentally not get as stressed out.

HCP: I like how you reframed the situation to one that has a more helpful tone and accurately reflects your situation. You may not be doing as much as you want, but we are working on ways to change that. And you are still engaged in the positive ways you mentioned. Do you notice any difference in your mood after thinking this through?

J: I feel less stressed. A little more relaxed, and hopefully I will get some sleep tonight.

HCP: Taking a moment to think it through and then reconsidering a way to reframe can be helpful. There are other ways, like relaxation, that can also help with your sleep. Let's talk about that.

RELAX AND REGULATE

Learning to self-regulate one's responses through relaxation techniques is a foundational skill for optimizing the management of pain and the use of medication. The body's stress response—which is not synonymous with pop culture's more general language of "being stressed"—is a physiological reaction to pain that leads to responses such as shallow breathing, increased heart rate, and muscle tension. These unhelpful responses can trigger forms of mental distress, such as worry and negativity. This alarm, useful in acute

or short-term pain, is not helpful with chronic pain, but without intervention it persists. Growing evidence suggests that relaxation techniques
can alter neural processing to reduce pain and cravings that may be present
with opioids (Dakwar & Levin, 2009; Zeidan et al., 2012)—so relaxation
provides another opportunity to retrain the brain and make it less susceptible
to unpleasant experiences.

For many people with chronic pain who also take opioids, the stress
response is stuck in the "on" position. A persistent heightened state of
arousal leads to shallow breathing and high levels of muscle tension becoming the norm rather than the exception. Unfortunately, this new pain-related
status quo increases pain sensitivity (Crettaz et al., 2013) and inflammation,
leading to physiological changes that make the presence of pain even more
detrimental to functioning.

The use of opioids and related concerns can lead to similar patterns of
anxiety and contribute to ongoing activation of the stress response. These
concerns include actual or anticipated increases in pain, when the next
dose of medication is scheduled, increasing use of PRN (i.e., pro re nata,
or as needed) medication options, how to balance activity engagement with
medication dosing, when the next doctor's appointment is scheduled, and
whether a loved one will be unhappy with medication use. Many people
who use opioids for pain management are familiar with these struggles and
more. Anxiety and distressing thoughts feed the stress response, increasing
pain and heightening unhelpful physical symptoms (Ploghaus et al., 2001).
Because of the relationship between the body's stress response and pain
and opioid processes, relaxation strategies provide an essential tool for
minimizing unwanted symptoms. Using relaxation techniques allows individuals to intervene and combat what has become the new baseline, leading
to reduced pain and lessening the power of opioids (Salamon et al., 2006).
By implementing the relaxation response, patients undo what may be years
of negative stress patterns and experience reduced pain, increased energy,
improved sleep, and decreased emotional distress (Kwekkeboom et al., 2010).
All of these outcomes have associated benefits, such as improving relationships and increasing social engagement. Individuals who use relaxation
effectively may also find a decreased need for opioid medications as their
pain and anxiety are better managed.

Steps to Self-Regulation

Relaxation is a portable and immediately accessible tool that should be
introduced to a patient as early as possible. While a variety of options may

be implemented, diaphragmatic or deep breathing is the cornerstone of all relaxation techniques. It is a brief and portable strategy that can be done anywhere, at any time, and usually without others becoming aware that it is being implemented. It involves breaths that are intentionally smoother, slower, and deeper than the breaths usually taken throughout the day. It is one of the easiest, most effective ways to decrease tension in the body. Through the practice of deep breathing, negative effects are undone—heart rate slows, muscle contractions loosen, and the mind is quieted.

Fortunately, the gateway to a better mental and physical state is easily accessible with a few basic steps. When a person focuses on breathing, their muscles and mind will relax automatically. Over time, this relaxed state will become the new normal: Individuals can change their physiology and be more in control of the typical stresses related to pain and opioid struggles.

Health care providers can teach patients to gain awareness of their current breathing and engage in diaphragmatic breathing, one of the most important approaches for pain and opioid management. The individual should take the following five steps to full breathing:

1. Establish good posture and a comfortable position—if on the go, even minor adjustments may help.
2. Place one hand on the chest and one hand on the abdomen. Notice whether you are chest breathing or belly breathing.
3. Slowly inhale through the nose for 3 to 4 seconds (count it!) and feel the abdomen expand.
4. Slowly and completely exhale through the mouth for 6 to 8 seconds.
5. Ideally continue for 3 to 5 minutes or longer. However, even five deep breaths will yield noticeable changes and benefits.

Patients should be encouraged to practice full breathing until they become comfortable with its use. It is important to engage the diaphragm for good breath efficiency, but rate is more important than depth of breath, which is why counting is key. For some people, this technique may come more easily than for others, but health care providers should stress the need for practice. A small subset of individuals (approximately 5%–10%) will experience heightened anxiety when they engage in relaxation training. This anxiety resolves with continued practice but can be understandably off-putting to patients, so providers should check in regularly during training to help monitor reactions and assist with acclimating to any new sensations. Many online resources and mobile apps, including low- and no-cost options, can be very helpful as complements to the health care provider and can facilitate regular practice.

A variety of additional strategies may assist with relaxation. Both breathing and these strategies can also be used to manage distress related to changes in opioid medication. Of note, various other options incorporate breathing techniques with movement-based approaches, including yoga and tai chi. Some commonly used relaxation techniques for chronic pain management include

- *progressive muscle relaxation* (PMR): PMR is a process of alternately contracting/tensing and relaxing muscles or muscle groups throughout the body (Turk & Monarch, 2002). PMR can be especially useful for individuals who prefer active physical engagement rather than relaxation options that favor stillness.

- *visualization and guided imagery*: Visualization is a process by which patients are encouraged to use all their senses to immerse themselves in a calming, vivid environment (Jamison, 1996). Guided imagery is another technique wherein the provider facilitates the patient focusing on mental images that evoke feelings of peace and relaxation (Chao & Ford, 2019; Fisher et al., 2018; Palermo, 2012). In guided imagery, the provider facilitates the patient focusing on mental images that evoke feelings of peace and relaxation. These strategies provide a point of focus away from pain and a means to decrease pain related thoughts and sensations.

- *autogenic training*: During this self-regulatory technique, individuals typically combine deep breathing, a calming visualization, and repetition of a phrase, promoting feelings of warmth and heaviness to induce a relaxed state (Kanji, 2000).

Ways to Use Relaxation

There are various ways to apply relaxation techniques and reap immediate benefits. Relaxation is widely used to help facilitate sleep. Because many individuals with chronic pain and opioid issues struggle with sleep, incorporating relaxation strategies into one's nightly routine can be valuable for calming the body and quieting the mind. Deep breathing can assist with falling asleep at night or returning to sleep after waking. By redirecting focus to the breath, individuals have a productive way to channel energy, rather than focusing on pain sensations or considering another dose of medication. However, health care providers may need to remind patients that while opioids may help with sleep onset due to sedation, they also cause sleep problems because they prevent users from reaching deep stages of sleep. Sleep quality is negatively impacted, and people feel less rested the next day.

Engagement for self-management strategies such as relaxation can be challenging. To achieve early success and patient buy-in, a health care provider may recommend that the patient combine relaxation with the following additional strategies:

- *drug deferral*: Relaxation strategies can be used to defer medication use. When a person experiences an increase in pain, stress, or both, the body's alarm system is on especially high alert. Intervening with a time delay for an evidence-based approach can be effective. When a patient expresses the desire to take a dose of medication, a health care provider can advise the person first to attempt an accessible relaxation option, such as deep breathing. This delay allows time to pass so that an impulsive reaction does not lead to medication use that is later regretted. In addition, using relaxation strategies can turn down the volume and regulate the heightened sensitivity in the body, potentially eliminating the individual's desire for the opioid after the brief delay. The provider approaches this strategy as a "just try it and see"—often patients are surprised at how helpful it is, and they skip the extra dose.

- *irritability flare*: Pain and changes in opioid use may increase irritability. When practiced regularly, relaxation strategies help to head off pain flares and aid in stress and opioid management. However, it is expected that pain and changes in opioid use may increase irritability.

- *sleep*: Sleep difficulties are common for individuals with pain, who may have trouble falling asleep and may wake often at night. Relaxation strategies such as breathing and visualization are accessible and effective strategies to improve sleep.

- *reduced dose companion*: For individuals on a fixed reduction of opioids, even when the plan is slow and reasonable, maintaining the tapering schedule may sometimes feel challenging mentally, physically, or both. Relaxation strategies are ideal for these instances.

The takeaway message for health care providers is that in the first patient meeting, it is useful to offer the five steps to breathe deep as a tool for the road. Relaxation can be used immediately to help retrain the body, aiding with muscle tension and other unhelpful symptoms of autonomic nervous system arousal. The autonomic nervous system can trigger the body's stress response as well as the relaxation response. Relaxation can be presented as an experiment, something to try until the next encounter just to see what happens—they might be surprised that even with this single tool they see decreases in pain as well as in opioid use.

ENGAGE IN ACTIVITIES SAFELY

For individuals with chronic pain who also use opioids, engaging in activities can be complicated. Some may tend to avoid activity altogether, whereas others may participate more than is safe for them. Many toggle between these extremes. Not doing enough and doing too much can both lead to negative consequences.

People with chronic pain withdraw from activities for a variety of reasons. They often worry that doing more will increase their pain or put them at risk of injury. When a pain-related issue is acute, avoiding activity on a short-term basis allows time for healing and restoration. Unfortunately, responding the same way to chronic pain not only is unhelpful but can be harmful. When pain is chronic, avoiding activity leads to physical deconditioning, a process by which individuals lose strength, stamina, and flexibility. They become more fatigued, may have spasms from tight muscles, and often gain weight, which adds strain to the body. Opioids may induce feelings of sedation or lethargy, and it becomes more comfortable to stay at home.

On the other hand, individuals who continue to engage in higher levels of activity, either on a regular basis or episodically, often find that their tendency to push through leads to pain flare-ups and other unwanted outcomes. Individuals may increase opioid use in an attempt to address pain resulting from physical engagement, may decrease activity entirely and be laid up for several days unable to do much of anything, or may experience a combination of these responses. Accomplishing a small goal in the moment is often at steep physical, emotional, and social costs. Avoiding or overdoing often leads to feelings of sadness, anxiety, guilt, or frustration regarding pain and opioid use as well as decreased feelings of control over life.

Although not often intuitive, one key strategy for managing pain and opioid use is to engage in activities thoughtfully on a regular basis. Engaging in a moderate amount of safe activity on a regular basis is one of the most important components of effective pain management. Activity helps to close the gate on increased pain and suffering and opens up more possibility for a meaningful life. However, because pain occurs with activity, a person may not believe that no damage is occurring.

Distinguishing Danger: How to Interpret Pain Signals

Chronic pain often changes how the nervous system works so that some patients feel more pain with less provocation, termed *central sensitization* (Woolf, 2011). This pain continually stimulates pathways, and because the human body is adaptable and experiences neuroplasticity, unhelpful changes can occur. When someone is in acute pain, the pain alarm serves a highly productive function: It helps identify pathology and a need for treatment and triggers protective behaviors that assist with the healing process. When pain persists, however, the pain system is chronically overexcited, often leading to central sensitization. The pain is still present and unpleasant, but the responses that were helpful for acute pain are counterproductive with chronic pain. In their seminal work, Butler and Moseley (2003) described pain as an output of the brain, which sends signals indicating danger even when that is not the case, harkening back to the neuromatrix of pain.

This situation presents one of the biggest challenges for individuals who experience and treat chronic pain: how to distinguish between a harm alarm that should be heeded and one that should not. Better understanding of central sensitization is critical, as the process has been identified in wide-ranging and common conditions such as low-back, neck, and shoulder pain; migraines; and fibromyalgia (Woolf, 2011). While central sensitization is not always present, these ideas are helpful when discussing whether to approach or to avoid activities. A health care provider can explain behavioral strategies as ways to calm an overactive nervous system. Because this idea does not imply disbelief, blame, or shame, patients are often more open to understanding the pain experience in this context.

Clinical Conundrum: Harm Alarm or Not?

On several occasions, Jim has discussed his fear about activities leading to increased pain, exacerbation of the problem, and reinjury. He frequently turns to rest and restriction of activity to address these concerns. The health care provider reviews the difference between pain as a symptom and pain as a condition as a way to encourage Jim to engage in healthy activity levels.

HEALTH CARE PROVIDER (HCP): There is a very common concern among people with persisting pain conditions that the pain is signaling some active damage or harm to the person, resulting in the person fearing they made their condition worse. Do you relate to this concern?

JIM (J): Absolutely. The last thing I want is for this to get any worse than it already is.

HCP: There are many reasons people continue to feel pain long after tissues have healed. Sometimes a structural issue continues to aggravate nerves, causing the pain sensation to generate, even though there isn't any immediate danger or new injury occurring.

J: Well, it feels like danger.

HCP: The persisting pain you feel is similar to the sensation of pain in a new injury. The difference is that new injuries are usually accompanied by new sensations in parts of the body other than where you feel persisting pain. The discomfort you feel in your low back is the same nerve aggravation that was seen on your MRIs over the past few years. The medical workup has been completed, and we know the physiological status. Sometimes when you overdo physical activities, the pain flares up and radiates into your right leg. That, too, is associated with the same nerve condition. Although it is painful, and I know that it is, it is not a new issue or a reason to head to the emergency room.

J: Well, how do I really know that?

HCP: That's a good question. Think back to a previous injury. You knew something was clearly wrong. To make it as simple as possible, how do you know you have a paper cut?

J. I feel a twinge when it happens, and yeah, it's something new in a place I don't usually feel that way.

HCP: And how do you respond?

J: I'll put pressure on it for a few seconds, then don't use my finger much for an hour or so, and it heals within a day or so.

HCP: Now, what if you felt that same twinge in your low back?

J: I wouldn't think anything of it because it's always acting that way.

HCP: Right, and that means it isn't an acute injury. Rather, the sensation is a symptom of your low back condition. So, what purpose does restricting activity and resting serve?

J: I don't know. It is just hard to do much when you are in pain. I know that avoiding things has made me feel worse. I'm getting weak, and I know it's not helping.

HCP: I would agree. The important takeaway is to know the difference between what is cause for concern and what is not. Even a pain flare-up is something you are familiar with and can get through without sounding the emergency alarms. A healthy level of activity for you means gradually increasing your limits to rebuild your body's strength and stamina for activity in general. We will keep figuring out how to do that together, figuring out where your pain tools, including opioids, fit in.

PACE THE RACE

Pacing is one important way to find balance between active periods and breaks so that one can stay engaged based on planning and not on pain. The key is to find balance so that activity is not an all-or-nothing, on-or-off proposition. Slowly adding activities based on patients' current functioning is a sensible way to start. For example, if an individual can currently walk for 10 minutes before beginning to feel uncomfortable, a health care provider can encourage them to start walking every day for 8 minutes. If someone is motivated to reconnect with friends, the provider might suggest scheduling a dinner date this week. Being reminded of how one feels after a walk or a dinner with friends can lead to increased openness to continue such activities.

Reconnecting with activities can be challenging given that predictability is often lacking in the lives of many people with chronic pain who use opioids. It is difficult to know how a person will feel, and the use of opioids are often linked with activity level. Pacing is the strongest way to achieve a more predictable life, which means less room for the physical and emotional ups and downs, which can be exhausting. Pacing, where time is the guide for activity engagement, allows for thoughtful and safe participation in many of the most important parts of life, such as taking a walk along the beach, playing in the park with grandchildren, going to an amusement park with friends, or tending to a vegetable garden. Instead of allowing the pain level to determine what the day looks like, a person can pace activities so that overdoing and underdoing are both avoided. Pacing helps to avoid the sawtooth up and down pattern in which surges of activity are followed by surges of rest; in essence, pacing allows for a plan-based rather than a pain-based or opioid-based life. Furthermore, pacing is the most crucial strategy in avoiding pain flare-ups and accompanying medication use.

Providers can introduce strategies for pacing directly. For example, a provider might recommend that the person find the baseline and boundaries, and stop before discomfort increases. The provider might ask, "How long can you engage in an activity before you become uncomfortable? Estimate the number of minutes you can safely do one of your regular activities (e.g., yardwork) and subtract 2 minutes—that is your 'up time.'" The provider might also recommend that the person take breaks: "Taking breaks allows you listen to your body, so it doesn't have to scream to get your attention! Plan your break times and use them to do another activity so that you can stay productive and engaged but allow rest for the needed area. For example, on your break from doing dishes you could sit and fold laundry, practice relaxation, or pay a bill online. Remember, by taking breaks you are helping yourself avoid pain flares and extended down time so you can be more efficient in the long run."

Pacing may also include breaking tasks into smaller, more manageable chunks and spreading them out over time. For example, instead of painting a room in one day, a person might use several days to complete the task. Instead of mowing the lawn in a single day and suffering the consequences for days after, a person might do the front yard today and the backyard tomorrow. While it can be frustrating to spread a task out and not get it accomplished at one time, implementing pacing means more productivity overall with less suffering—a winning combination.

ENJOY MORE

It is not uncommon for individuals with pain who use opioids to have lost many enjoyable things in their lives. Everything can feel like it is determined by pain and opioids, and that impacts even those areas of life that people usually favor, such as hobbies and spending time with friends and family. In addition, because they are often focused on bigger issues, such as receiving a more satisfying diagnosis or pursuing medical treatments, people with pain who use opioids may not feel that they can enjoy or appreciate the benefit of pleasant activities. Furthermore, the use of opioids may have negatively affected the person's relationships, making isolation more appealing than socialization. Benefits of activities that involve others include fostering friendships and deepening family connections. However, people who use opioids may feel judged harshly, even by those with whom they are close, and may thus want to avoid interactions with others. They may feel that social interactions are not fun, that they are too irritable, or that no one understands them. If they plan activities around pain levels and opioid use, they may feel hesitant to make plans, lacking confidence in their ability to follow through. The lack of pleasant activities decreases quality of life and often increases low mood. Without positive inputs, individuals have more opportunities for negative mood and experiences.

The potential benefits of engaging in pleasant activities include the following:

- improved mood and self-esteem (Gardner & Oei, 1981; Grosscup & Lewinsohn, 1980)
- increased socialization (Lewinsohn et al., 1978)
- enhanced attention and concentration (Logsdon et al., 2007)
- positive distraction (Stevens & Lane, 2001)
- added sense of purpose and direction (Wilson & Murrell, 2004)

Engaging in pleasant activities is an effective technique for reducing distress in many people (Ekers et al., 2008). Increasing pleasurable activities and improving low mood can help close the door on pain and can decrease desire for opioids. Increasing enjoyable activities can be categorized as an external distraction, which is a powerful source of attentional diversion that can mediate the anxiety that contributes to reduced pain tolerance (Arntz et al., 1994; James & Hardardottir, 2002; Johnson et al., 1998). Since individuals have a finite amount of attention that they can give, focusing on something that they genuinely find interesting and enjoyable makes less space available to focus on pain or opioids. Given that, the provider should encourage the development of activities that are personally enjoyable for each patient. The activities may vary across individuals, so health care providers should never make assumptions about what may be fun or not. For example, one person may enjoy going to the beach, but another may find the sun and sand annoying and aversive. One person may enjoy the country and camping, but another may find that setting unappealing due to bugs or lack of technology. A provider should help each patient identify what they find enjoyable, with the patient exploring and spelling out the details of intended activities.

It is also important for a health care provider to inquire about and consider the role that opioids may have played in various pleasant activities. Someone may have used opioids to engage in or assist with recovery from unpaced activities (i.e., overdoing it, or exceeding their current tolerance for that activity). Or some of the pleasant activities they once engaged in placed them around people who use opioids recreationally. In these situations, the provider can use any of the following strategies:

- *extend appreciation*: "I am so grateful that you trusted me enough to share this information about these potential triggering people and places. I know that was not easy for you."

- *suggest external support*: "Since your brother encourages your opioid-related changes and enjoys animals like you do, perhaps he could join you the next time you volunteer."

- *brainstorm concrete alternatives*: "Let's discuss the strategies that you have in your toolbox now that could be used so that you either avoid these scenarios or feel confident in how to engage. For example, if we know these individuals work on certain days, then you can set up your volunteer schedule on other days. We can also take a more assertive approach for how to clearly articulate how you will manage these scenarios."

- *rehearse*: "One thing we can do is role-play these situations so you have experience with exactly what to say. We know that rehearsing effective responses is better than simply talking about what you might do."

PROBLEM-SOLVING

When discussing pleasant activities, it is important to remember that just because someone wants to and is willing to do something, they may not be able to, especially if resources are restricted. People may feel discouraged about not doing things the way they used to or the way they want to. They may become negative toward themselves; this negativity is unhelpful and can reduce engagement.

Often, a person may need to consider alternative ways to engage in activities to account for limiting factors (e.g., physical, financial). A health care provider can help the patient plan how the activity might happen and identify areas in which creativity or flexibility may be needed for the execution. For example, engaging in certain sports, such as golf or tennis, may have a high price tag. A provider can take time to discuss how the individual may realistically reconsider engaging in the activity. For example, might they join a peer who is a member at a golf club so they do not have to pay greens fees? Could they go to a low-cost driving range for practice? Is there a community tennis court where they could hit balls or play at certain times for minimal cost? When determining a plan, the provider and patient should discuss other logistics as well, such as how the person will travel to and from the activity, who might join them, and when it is reasonable to participate (e.g., day(s) of week, time(s) of day).

A health care provider can also help patients to explore modified and creative options for how they can still access the pleasure of the things they used to enjoy, but in a different way. For example, a patient may say that they used to enjoy fishing but now can't do it; the last time they tried they were laid up for days and ended up taking a bunch of meds just to get through. A provider might ask the following questions:

- "What was it that you enjoyed most about fishing?" It may have been being outside, the people with whom they frequently fished, or the quiet that it brought. When planning the modification, it is helpful for the provider to understand the meaning that the activity held for the patient.

- "Are you willing to teach others to fish?" Sharing the hobby with others, including with someone in the family, may be a less physically intense but more meaningful pathway to reconnect with the sport and a way to increase self-esteem through sharing knowledge and experience.

- "Have you ever used a gaming system?" Advanced graphics and accessories allow for modified activity within the home in an adapted but fun way that can be done solo or with friends.

- "Do you have other ideas for reconnecting to the essence of the activity?" If the social aspect was most meaningful, the patient may find another way to access others. If being outdoors is a gap in the person's life at present, the provider may help the person to explore other ways to capture that experience.

Clinical Conundrum: Engaging in Pleasant Activities

Given Jim's tendency to avoid activities outside of work, it is important that the health care provider brings to light what he used to enjoy doing as well as how to engage in activities that are both necessary and meaningful. The provider engages Jim in discussion of how to approach an activity of interest to him.

HEALTH CARE PROVIDER (HCP):   You mentioned before that it was important to you to pitch in around the house and participate in more social gatherings, but right now those activities feel like too much. Let's explore how you might start. Which activity do you want to start with, assuming it's a small step?

JIM (J):   I know I should get out more. My wife is always inviting me to different things, and it's fun some of the time when I go, but since I don't know how I'll feel, I say no a lot.

HCP: What is it about going out with your wife that you enjoy?

J: Well, she likes it, and I like going out, talking to our friends, the change in scenery. I just don't like when it's all night, like that time they went on a party bus ride. After a couple hours, I'm ready to go home.

HCP: So, it sounds like you do enjoy going out with your wife and friends, but it would work better if your activity was time limited. Perhaps you could suggest activities that would fall within a time frame that you think is reasonable given your limitations, as a starting point.

J: Going out for a couple of hours seems to work well. So going out to dinner with other couples or even going to a movie with my wife could work.

HCP: Would you consider those small steps?

J: Yeah, those are both pretty manageable.

HCP: So, how would you set this up?

J: I'll talk to my wife about getting some people together for dinner out. She would probably like that I'm actually suggesting something for once.

HCP: This could be an opportunity for you to connect with her also, since you said things had been a bit disconnected between you. And this sounds like a realistic goal. Now let's map out more of the details to make it SMART.

REINFORCING STRATEGIES

When possible, a health care provider should connect what the patient discusses spontaneously with the behavioral strategies that are taught. For instance, when reviewing homework, if a patient reports improved mood or increased energy, the provider might see an opportunity to help the person identify what they did to create this outcome. Asking about the action taken by the individual leaves no question about self-efficacy—this outcome did not "just happen" by chance or coincidence, but rather the individual made certain choices and generated this outcome. Empowering people to believe in themselves and their agency in improving pain and opioid-related status is central to treatment. Repetition of skills through routine, real-world practice demonstrates effectiveness that they can see; in addition, helping patients connect their behavioral changes to their reported progress helps reinforce patients' understanding of the biopsychosocial nature of pain as well as strengthens their trust in the utility of nonopioid approaches. Over the course of treatment, patients develop a greater appreciation for their important part in managing pain and opioids through continual practice, problem solving, and feedback. The health care provider takes on the role of consultant and teammate, offering support as needed. The provider also functions as a mindset coach, facilitating each person's understanding and ability to persevere despite pain and opioid-related obstacles that may arise.

CONCLUSION

When applied on a consistent basis, the strategies presented in this chapter create the backbone for effective management of pain and opioids to minimize fluctuations and maximize control. The implementation of these strategies will ensure that patients obtain optimal benefit across treatments—the use of medications, movement-based therapies, and other treatment modalities will be optimized when self-managed behavioral options are the foundation. Incorporating even one strategy at a time can prove helpful; as success breeds confidence and openness, other tools can be added with cumulative benefit.

8 ADDRESS COMMON BARRIERS

There is a dearth of research regarding how best to support individuals with pain who are making adjustments to opioid medications, in part due to knowledge gaps between the letter of clinical recommendations and the reality of clinical practice. In their examination of patients' perspectives during opioid deprescribing, Frank et al. (2016) noted that strong psychosocial support from friends, family, and health care providers can serve as one potential facilitator for success. The benefits of support are similar to feedback from patients with chronic pain regarding use of pain self-management practices (Bair et al., 2009). Strong communication and trusting relationships with health care providers can aid in elucidating barriers and strengths when instituting behavioral interventions (Chipidza et al., 2015; Greene et al., 2016; Ha & Longnecker, 2010; Sherman et al., 2018). Whereas Chapter 7 included specific strategies to manage pain and opioid analgesics, this chapter carefully examines the challenges that may arise when implementing these approaches and includes strategies to best address those challenges. Providers should expect inconsistencies in patient implementation of the strategies introduced,

https://doi.org/10.1037/0000209-009
Chronic Pain and Opioid Management: Strategies for Integrated Treatment,
by J. L. Murphy and S. Rafie

as patients often need regular reminders about the ways in which prescribed behavioral interventions can turn down the volume on pain and empower them to rely less on opioids.

FLARE-UPS

Pain flare-ups can be among the biggest barriers for implementing behavioral pain medicine strategies. These actual or anticipatory pain flares commonly lead to increased use of opioid analgesics and thus are particularly important to address in integrated treatment. While it is unlikely that patients can eliminate pain flares completely, they can rely on various techniques to reduce and manage them. Since fluctuations in pain and the need for opioids can be one of the greatest frustrations for individuals, health care providers should remind them of ways to alleviate feelings of helplessness and instill those of self-efficacy.

One of the primary reasons to institute the behavioral techniques on a consistent basis is to minimize the occurrence of flare-ups. Strategies include

- *planning and pacing activities*: Avoiding underdoing and overdoing allows an individual to take control of pain and opioids by increasing predictability in daily life.

- *getting sufficient sleep each night*: Without proper rest, patients are primed to experience more pain, frustration, and associated opioid use during the day (Moldofsky, 2001; Raymond et al., 2004).

- *altering diet*: Patients can avoid foods that increase inflammation (e.g., processed meats, sugary drinks, white bread, pasta) and increase consumption of those that are anti-inflammatory (e.g., raw nuts, fish, vegetables, fruit; Maroon et al., 2010; Seaman, 2012).

- *using relaxation techniques early and often*: The more relaxation is used, the faster patients will be able to reprogram their brains and bodies to minimize those unhelpful danger signals and stop using opioids as their only de-stressor.

- *circumventing triggers*: Instead of engaging in scenarios that are known to turn up stress and tension, leading to increased pain and opioid use, individuals can refrain from triggering situations whenever possible or enter prepared with relaxation techniques and social support at hand.

When pain increases do occur, individuals have a variety of options to manage the presence of flare-ups using the following strategies:

- *taking a break*: This does not mean avoiding everything but rather pausing to use active strategies such as relaxation techniques to gain control over one's body and mind.

- *using water*: Gentle movement in a warm pool or the use of hot water in a shower or tub can be particularly therapeutic in the midst of a pain increase.

- *distracting with an interest*: Individuals can find something that is both engaging and calming to take their mind to another place and lower stress and muscle tension.

- *talking to someone*: Individuals can find someone to connect with on the phone, online, or in person.

- *spending energy wisely*: Focusing limited energy on doing something that will be helpful in decreasing negative impacts and restoring homeostasis is better than going down a dark path of unhelpful thoughts related to pain and opioids.

NOT ENOUGH MOTIVATION

Individuals with pain may need motivational enhancement strategies throughout the treatment process, particularly when they need to handle opioid-related concerns. Many people who have an overreliance on substances feel an ambivalence or resistance to beginning treatment as well as staying the course once they have decided to make a treatment attempt. When implementing behavioral techniques, it may be helpful for the individual and health care provider to return to a conversation about the negative consequences that have resulted from opioid use and that may have affected loved ones, employment, finances, or the patient's emotional and physical health. Circling back to what brought individuals with chronic pain and opioid struggles into treatment can be a helpful way to refocus on why strategies for management are important. This discussion typically goes hand in hand with specifying the benefits of reducing or discontinuing use. Providers should allow patients to elucidate their vision of how life might improve if opioids were not on center stage. Even individuals who are less enthusiastic about making changes to their opioid regimen can typically identify the costs that have come with the medications and the ways that life would improve without them.

Using open-ended questions stimulates the conversation when individuals are resistant to remaining in treatment, implementing the suggested tools, or making changes to one's opioid regimen:

- "How do you think that reducing your use of opioids would affect your ability to reach your personal goals?"
- "How might decreasing your use of opioids change your relationships?"
- "If you reduce your reliance on opioids, what changes would you be happy to see in your life?"

If they have already begun to decrease opioids and are wavering, this conversation is an opportunity to openly discuss their experience and concerns:

- "How has your life been different since you began decreasing your opioids?"
- "What are you most concerned about right now?"
- "Have you received feedback from anyone else since initiating the slow taper?"

To help patients remain engaged in treatment, providers should express understanding and normalize their changing thoughts and emotions. They should reassure individuals that behavioral changes are difficult to make (Kelly & Barker, 2016), especially when they involve a potential increase in temporary discomfort that may result from increased movement or decreased opioid dosage.

Clinical Conundrum: Pain Flare Leads to Losing Motivation

Jim has begun to pace activities at home, especially more enjoyable things around the house, but with his usual full-time work schedule, he noted near-daily flare-ups. He has managed these flare-ups for 2 weeks by reducing activities and relying on medication and rest as his primary pain management tools. The health care provider reviews psychoeducation to help with pain flare-up prevention and management while focusing on enhancing his motivation for change.

HEALTH CARE PROVIDER (HCP):   Pacing work activities is harder for you than pacing leisure, so we will spend some time developing a realistic pacing plan for your work activities later today. That is key to minimizing increases in pain. But remember, what you do after the flare-up starts is also very important. Medicating and rest won't get you far, considering you'll end up in the same place later. What tools that we've discussed might be worthwhile to try when you get home from work?

JIM (J): I should go for a walk, and I need to use the breathing. The breathing always helps some.

HCP: Great ideas. Something active may help with how your body feels and to clear your mind, while breathing also eases both body and mind. You're aware of what you could do, but how are you feeling as far as motivation? You said that you had returned to the old way of dealing with the pain, like resting and using opioids to get you through the day. I'm curious if you've had any positive changes in your life since you first reduced your dosage.

J: It's been good to be a bit more active and get along better with my wife. I lost a few pounds, too, which was nice.

HCP: Those sound like important positives. Weren't those all related to your initial goals we discussed?

J. They were, yeah. I wanted to feel better physically, be able to do more, and work on my marriage.

HCP: It's not uncommon for people to have a bump in the road on their way to their goals. How do you feel about continuing toward those goals, rather than on the path you've taken these past couple weeks? What would you like to do?

J: I'll keep working on it. It all sort of piled up quickly with my job, but I can work on it again. Can we meet again in a couple weeks to check in?

HCP: Yes, great idea.

PATIENT RESISTANCE

Many obstacles may present over the course of treatment. Some hurdles are experienced by the patient (e.g., setbacks in progress, psychosocial stressors, change in work demands), but often the challenges are experienced by the provider, in the form of pushback from the patient regarding treatment recommendations. The most commonly resisted tools are cognitive reframing, relaxation training, and behavioral activation. The following sections include sample statements from patients as well as suggested responses for providers.

Resistance to Rethinking

Even when introducing a focus on cognitions, it is important for a provider to offer an explanation about how a person's thinking can impact their pain experience and opioid use. The reality is that it can be challenging for individuals to consider the role of their own thoughts despite confirmation that there are no concerns about blame or causality. Health care providers may hear objections that sound something like the following:

- "It is not all in my head."
- "Opioids are the only thing that help, changing my thoughts doesn't change that!"
- "This isn't about thinking—no one understands."

The content of these thoughts is less important than reminding patients of a few things:

- "I believe you! I know that you have pain every day, that it is frustrating and unpleasant and not your fault. That is our baseline."

- "As we discussed, science shows us the undeniable brain-based power that these thoughts can have on our pain experience and our level of stress, things that often fuel opioid use."

- "The more that we engage in these unhelpful thoughts, the more control we give pain. The good news is that we can be more aware of these unhelpful thoughts that do not serve us and make changes so that our life improves."

When individuals have acknowledged these ideas, the health care provider can revisit skills for adapting cognitions to be more beneficial.

Resistance to Relaxation

Relaxation is perhaps the most accessible tool that can be offered to assist those with pain and opioid issues, but that does not mean that it is always easily incorporated. While some take to it immediately, others voice objections:

- "I'm not stressed. I do plenty to relax and don't see the point of this."
- "I tried a couple of times, but it doesn't do anything."
- "It always makes me fall asleep, but I don't see it helping with pain or opioids."

Providers can use the following pointers to help address common barriers that patients may present:

- "Sometimes it does not come easily—it took a long time for your stress meter to get stuck 'on.' It takes some practice to help retrain the body."

- "Biofeedback may be a way to help you better see how your body decompresses when you use relaxation. If you are interested, we can explore it as another way to help with learning self-regulation."

- "It can be a useful option to help initiate sleep but can also help with decreased muscle tension and changing opioid usage by combatting intense situations. Perhaps try using it outside of bedtime to see what happens."

Resistance to Activity

Engaging in activity, especially when physically painful, is often the biggest source of resistance. It may take repeated explanations of the chronic pain fear-avoidance cycle for people to feel safe doing more. For some, activation may need to come before motivation—if they are willing to take a small step, reinforcement follows. Common complaints include the following:

- "It hurts too much to move."
- "I actually walked all day with my family at the zoo, and all it did was lead to more opioids and more time on the sofa."
- "I thought about going for a walk, but I really don't like sweating and would rather be doing something else."

The following suggestions can be useful in addressing concerns:

- "I realize it may seem counterintuitive, but moving just a little bit more is actually the best thing you can do for yourself. Motion is lotion for the joints and helps to decrease inflammation."

- "Remember pacing? It is great that you went to the zoo, but it sounds as if, instead of taking breaks, you went full force all day and suffered a major pain flare-up. Let's discuss how you might have approached things differently and avoided that."

- "It is so important to choose activities we enjoy. Since you prefer the cool air, perhaps you could go for a walk at the mall, a museum, or the aquarium with a friend."

For many, getting going can be the most challenging part, but if they wait until they "feel like" moving, the time may not come, and another day will go by without this helpful treatment. Research shows that engaging in activity changes can induce positive feelings immediately (Mazzucchelli et al., 2010): Sometimes we must choose to do, and the "good" chemicals in the brain that reinforce doing the same behavior again will follow.

Health care providers can also remind patients that small choices can make a big difference over time:

- "Instead of taking the closest parking space, choose one that is a bit farther away."

- "While watching TV, do stretches or lunges, or use hand weights while seated to move your arms."

- "Take the stairs instead of the elevator. The difference in calorie burning and joint flexibility matters."

- "Go to the gym, YMCA, community center, or senior center for activities like swimming or adaptive gentle yoga, often seated!"

Clinical Conundrum: Talk About Resistance

Tired and irritable, Jim communicates to his provider that he is unsure if the skills are working. He discusses his use of activity scheduling, cognitive reframing, and relaxation techniques and notes they have had limited benefit. The health care provider responds with reminders about the approaches while gently challenging beliefs related to reliance on opioids and encouraging adaptation of skills into practice.

JIM (J):   I'm not that stressed, and I tried some things. It's just that opioids are the only thing that seem to help me, and I'm used to them, so I take my pill and relax on the couch at night after work.

HEALTH CARE PROVIDER (HCP):   It sounds like you are looking for more benefits, but you're focused more on taking medications, which I know doesn't require the same amount of involvement. However, when we began talking, you shared the many ways your life wasn't what you wanted it to be and said you wanted more options.

J: I know. I just don't know that they work, and I'm too exhausted to do them a lot of the time.

HCP: We discussed the breathing exercises that can be a useful option to help initiate sleep, reduce muscle tension, and change opioid usage by combatting intense situations. Our thoughts can open the gates to pain and distress, things that often fuel opioid use. And we know that deconditioning from avoidance is something you wanted to change. You also had a walking goal you had set. Tell me why you decided to stop that.

J: My whole day at work is spent on my feet, walking from one place to another. I'm already avoiding the walks at work as much as I can, so why would I go for a walk once I'm home or even in the morning when I could be relaxing?

HCP: We know physical tools are an important part of taking care of your overall health. Perhaps, for you, the focus is more on restorative activities, like yoga or stretching. It's great that you are sharing your thoughts with me as we go, so we can figure out a plan that suits you best. A plan is only valuable if it is realistic. Let's uncover your motivation and get back to basics.

TRIGGERS

Another way to decrease downward spirals precipitated by pain and opioids is to minimize triggers. Raising awareness of situations that may trigger increased pain and use of opioids is an important step in setting up patients for success. Work with individuals to identify the sources in the pain and opioid world that may lead to exacerbations. While the person is sharing, prompt them for details—the more specific a picture, the more likely it is that a trigger can be avoided or managed effectively:

- "What situation triggered an increase in pain or the desire to use opioids?"
- "What were you thinking or feeling at the time?"
- "What action did you take?"
- "What happened? Tell me the positive and the negative."

The responses to these inquiries can help the provider better understand what specific steps to take to help patients minimize the triggers. For example, a patient may recognize that when her in-laws come over for their weekly visit, she tends to spend hours cleaning the day before, which often leads to increased pain and additional use of PRN opioid medications. The provider can help by discussing how she can better incorporate pacing. If she spread out cleaning tasks throughout the week, she would feel less pressure before the visit. Perhaps she could ask her children to assist with cleaning chores. Additional examination of the thoughts that accompany these times might reveal that she is being overly critical and that extensive cleaning is unnecessary. By using pacing, enlisting the help of others, and being gentler on herself, in the upcoming weeks she may find that she does not take any extra opioid medications before or during these visits.

Patients are more successful with problem-solving the issues that inevitably arise when providers openly discuss obstacles and routes forward. It is important for health care providers to remember that individuals who have chronic pain and use opioids face fluctuations in their pain experience and their attitudes toward medications. Positive reinforcement of successes and reminders about strengths help to foster trust and collaboration. Finally, providers should remind patients that while each strategy is helpful in addressing pain and opioid management, the person's chance of having better days and outcomes is multiplied when the strategies are used together.

Clinical Conundrum: Talk About Triggers

Jim has high levels of stress driving into work each day, resulting from traffic and time constraints. This stress leads to increased pain upon arrival, mental strain from the drive that launches a tension headache, the use of additional opioids to "get through"—which takes the edge off but means more sedation, and decreased productivity overall at work. The health care provider facilitates a problem-solving discussion to identify alternative plans for managing the triggering situation that may decrease the potency of the trigger.

HEALTH CARE PROVIDER (HCP):   It seems the daily commute is a clear source of stress and tension for you, and it makes for a less-than-ideal start to the day.

JIM (J):   It's like that every day. I hate it.

HCP: Perhaps leaving earlier would decrease traffic flow and allow more breathing room so you feel less rushed. What else might help?

J: I usually listen to loud music during the ride. In a way, it is a stress reliever, but I've also noticed that it can crank up my tension. Based on what we've talked about, I guess I could use some of the time to play my relaxation audio file and practice those techniques.

HCP: That's another great option. Anything else?

J: Well, a guy at work mentioned carpooling, asked me if I was interested. There's a few people in my area who do that. I don't really want to be around other people in the morning, but it would mean I had to drive less often. I could do something as a passenger, like listen to music or the relaxation stuff, or even read. Would also save money on gas, so that could make sense.

HCP: Another solid option. Let's discuss these and determine a plan for moving ahead.

CONCLUSION

It is wonderful to have empirically supported behavioral approaches to pain and opioid management, but they matter very little if patients are unwilling or unable to engage with the helpful approaches that are offered. Health care providers are often faced with ambivalence and resistance toward change, particularly behavioral adjustments, and that is normal and expected. These barriers in clinical care must be addressed as often as they are encountered. When health care providers have strategies to manage the obstacles before they come up, they can feel prepared to handle even the most challenging situations.

9 MONITOR AND MANAGE SYMPTOMS

Managing pain and opioids is often highly complex because of the presence of psychiatric and medical comorbidities as well as challenging psychosocial circumstances. For the population comanaging chronic pain and opioids, therefore, it is particularly important to appropriately recognize any symptoms that may arise related to these multimorbidities or changes in opioid regimens. Opioids can mask issues that may not have been appropriately identified or addressed previously, such as anxiety-related disorders. Despite efforts to support rational and slowly paced opioid reductions, some patients may experience increased anticipation related to withdrawal symptoms, which must be addressed. It is critical for the health care provider to stay connected and aligned with patients during this process, walk them through unfamiliar experiences in emotional and physical domains, and continue ongoing treatment planning based on any concerns. Importantly, symptoms and signs that were denied or not apparent at the outset of treatment may emerge over time, suggesting the presence of opioid use disorder (OUD) and indicating that further evaluation and triage are necessary. Some patients who are implementing behavioral strategies for pain and opioid

https://doi.org/10.1037/0000209-010
Chronic Pain and Opioid Management: Strategies for Integrated Treatment,
by J. L. Murphy and S. Rafie

management require additional support, and it is important that a provider follow them closely throughout the process.

REDUCTION EXPECTATIONS

When considering making a change to opioid medications, it is recommended that possible fears and previous reduction experiences be explored early in the process. Normalizing experiences and creating realistic expectations can be powerful tools for minimizing unhelpful thinking that can accompany novel approaches to pain management and to changes in medication regimens. Individuals who have been taking opioids regularly, particularly for prolonged periods, should anticipate a period of adjustment psychologically. For many, medication has gained a prominence in their lives that is not fully recognized. It may be the first thing individuals think about upon waking, activities may be organized around times when medications are administered, and bedtime behaviors may be affected—in essence, the medications control their behavior and lives. According to the literature, the most common fears about opioid reduction are increased pain and experiencing withdrawal symptoms.

OPIOID REDUCTION: MANAGING BODY AND MIND

Since symptoms are variable and can arise at any point during the opioid tapering process, individuals should be monitored closely throughout so that emerging issues are attended to as soon as possible. Health care providers should be aware of preexisting concerns that are managed on a long-term basis, such as Type 2 diabetes or depression, as increases in pain and changes in opioid use can have physical effects that impact how these conditions are experienced and managed. For example, a patient with diabetes who is not adequately managing pain based on the suggested behavioral skills and experiences pain flare-ups may resort to overeating as a way to cope with discomfort or stress. This response could lead to increases in blood sugar and insulin needs. Conversely, for someone with Type 2 diabetes who is fully engaged in treatment, behavioral activation may lead to decreased blood sugar, which can cause a decreased need for insulin; without proper monitoring and awareness, the accompanying hypoglycemia can become an acute medical issue. Individuals outside the medical field may feel less prepared and less comfortable addressing the potential relationship between behavioral changes and various health conditions. At a minimum, however, all health care professionals should encourage open and ongoing communication from the patient regarding any changes and ensure that the medical team is adequately engaged.

Symptoms related to reductions in the use of opioids must also be closely monitored and reported to the medical team. Physical withdrawal symptoms are particularly significant concerns for patients, and although thoughtful and slowly paced tapering plans minimize these symptoms, they can still occur. At times, medications such as clonidine may be prescribed to reduce physical discomfort (Gowing et al., 2016). As reviewed in Chapter 1, the most common symptoms of withdrawal include the following:

- nausea and vomiting
- sweating, fever, or chills
- restlessness or anxiety
- rapid heart rate
- increased pain
- trouble sleeping
- agitation (physical and mental; World Health Organization, 2009)

It is important to remind individuals that withdrawal symptoms can occur when the body has become used to something, including caffeine and nicotine. It is helpful to include a medical provider in the discussion when possible so they can evaluate symptom severity and determine if an adjustment to the rate of taper is indicated. As has been noted, the literature suggests that slow tapers minimize signs and symptoms of withdrawal (U.S. Department of Health and Human Services, 2019a).

While physical concerns may arise, it is more likely that changes in emotional status will occur, and these changes are generally less anticipated or adequately addressed. Opioid changes can be associated with the emergence or exacerbation of psychiatric symptoms for a number of reasons. Opioids may have served as a global numbing agent that masked a variety of issues, including mood-related symptoms. As a result, reductions in opioid analgesics can lead to an unveiling of complaints that have previously been unrecognized or not fully realized. For example, for those with posttraumatic stress disorder (PTSD), opioids may have numbed anxious symptoms and dulled cognitive processes. They may have declined other appropriate treatments for PTSD, such as trauma-focused therapy or pharmaceuticals, preferring the use of opioid analgesics as a means to avoid addressing difficult topics more directly. As opioid dose is reduced, health care providers are likely to see patients experience increased anxiety and other symptoms related to the underlying untreated psychiatric issue. At times, patients may have been self-medicating for a disorder such as PTSD for so many years that they have never presented for treatment or received a diagnosis. This situation can make things even more complicated and necessitates a thorough evaluation, ideally by a mental health clinician who can determine the person's history, symptom presence and pattern, functional impacts, and treatment needs. Throughout the course of care, the health care team should be prepared to visit and revisit a biopsychosocial framework to address treatment needs appropriately.

It may be difficult to determine whether symptoms such as increased agitation, restlessness, and anxiety are related to opioid reduction, the underlying mental health condition, or perhaps a combination of both. Several steps can be helpful in the process. First, typical withdrawal symptoms should be addressed with medical measures as indicated (e.g., clonidine). Appropriate medical interventions may not only quiet the physiological symptoms but also may provide room to discuss potential psychological concerns. For individuals who have been disconnected with or unwilling to address a mental health issue directly, it can be helpful for a health care professional to normalize the role of opioids in their experience up to now. This is not about blaming patients or making them feel accused of misusing opioids; rather, the conversation should be a supportive and empathic interaction in which individuals feel understood and comfortable being open about how opioids may have helped them manage their feelings. The provider should also remind patients of the potential dangers of self-medicating and the benefits of addressing emotional issues more directly.

In some instances, it can be useful for the health care professional to draw a direct comparison between the unhelpful role of avoidance in maintaining both chronic pain and emotional distress. Many individuals respond to their pain by avoiding people, places, and things. They decrease activities to avoid increasing pain and to avoid difficult social experiences. However, these behaviors generally do not lead to better quality of life and functioning; rather, they perpetuate a cycle of increased pain, disability, and isolation. A similar process can be seen for individuals struggling with mental health issues. They want to avoid the pain that accompanies dealing directly with issues such as depression or anxiety, and they pursue various forms of self-medication to do so. Unfortunately, not addressing these symptoms and their underlying causes directly will likely lead to greater suffering in the long term. If patients have benefitted from managing their pain in a more direct way, they may more easily see the potential pluses of treating emotional issues in a more direct manner.

Since turning or returning to opioids in the face of psychological challenges is not uncommon, it is important to clarify why pain and significant emotional stressors should be managed in parallel.

Clinical Conundrum: Addressing Reduction-Related Concerns

Jim began a slow-paced opioid taper several weeks ago, and it has been going well. However, the health care provider receives a call one morning in which Jim reports that he did not sleep well last night and has felt more agitated and anxious today. He presents for an appointment later the same day to follow up on his concerns. The health care provider actively listens, assuages fears, provides concrete options, and stays connected with the patient.

HEALTH CARE PROVIDER (HCP):   I received your message today, and I understand that you have not been at your best. Tell me what happened in the past few days.

JIM (J):   I've been going through the process with the medication change, and the past few days have been rough, but last night I couldn't get a wink of sleep. I've been on edge and not feeling well physically or mentally today.

HCP: It sounds like the increased restlessness overnight left you feeling uneasy and set you up for increased pain sensitivity and irritability today. Since you are generally doing very well, it makes sense to actively examine and address what is happening in your life before we make any reactive changes to your medication. The good news is that we have strategies to manage these issues, so we will discuss those and continue to track how you are feeling. Tell me what else has been going on recently for you?

J: My daughter got accepted into a program that would cost us a lot of money, and we've already been barely making it with expenses. I'm careful with money and don't overspend, but it would be nice to save some for a rainy day. So that's been on my mind since last week, and it kept me up the night she got the news.

HCP: So let's discuss the unexpected stressors that surfaced in the last few days and how we can address the anxiety they are causing. Remember that we have learned that opioids have a sedating effect in the evening and that they allow you to close off to mental chatter more easily. As the dose decreases, we need to be sure to implement the tools that we have. If you have difficulty again tonight, instead of watching a political show that is stimulating, would you be willing to try a breathing exercise?

J: I can do that. That was helping for stress before.

HCP: You also may want to examine your thoughts about the stressors to be sure you aren't at extremes, which can be unhelpful. Sometimes, talking to your wife or writing down your thoughts might also be helpful as a way of expressing yourself before you go to bed. And of course, just as you did this time, call me any time you have concerns so that we can troubleshoot.

HIGH ALERT

Two clinical concerns should be monitored with vigilance, as they can be matters of life and death. First, it is critical that the health care provider stay attuned to the possible presence of OUD. As discussed previously, increased agitation and restlessness are common withdrawal symptoms and do not necessarily indicate OUD. For example, Jim's symptoms were manageable during the day and were interfering primarily in the evening. They also interfered with sleep onset and maintenance after he had received some anxiety-provoking news. In similar cases, a health care provider may remind the patient that some level of sleep disruption is not unusual during opioid changes but will decrease with physical acclimation. This type of education may help decrease the patient's catastrophizing. In the case example, Jim finds using full breathing techniques when he is initiating sleep helps significantly and reports no further issues, but a patient who reveals a different clinical picture requires different follow-up. For example, a patient who is reducing her opioids may share that she has been unable to manage anxiety despite using recommended strategies and has not gone to work in days; she may tearfully admit that she purchased medication from a neighbor in a moment of desperation. For this patient, an OUD evaluation should be done because her response to the tapering effort suggests a possible diagnosis. Because she is making poor and risky choices in response to stress, buprenorphine-naloxone may very well be in order and most therapeutic.

Second, emerging data suggest that the period following taper is one of increased risk for patients, indicating the need for follow-up (Hundley et al., 2018; Oliva et al., 2020). Although this is a time where treatment is typically considered successfully completed, providers are encouraged to think of cessation as another step in treatment that requires ongoing monitoring. In a large observational evaluation in the Veterans Health Administration, Oliva et al. (2020) found that patients were at greater risk of death from overdose or suicide after stopping opioid treatment, with increased risk the longer patients had been treated before stopping. Furthermore, the data suggested individuals who have reduced opioids may be especially vulnerable in the first 1 to 3 months following tapering. While such an evaluation should not be considered causal, the importance of taking steps such as routine follow-up care to mitigate risks whenever opioids are stopped is strongly supported (Berna et al., 2015). Another potential unintended consequence of tapering may be that patients may feel abandoned. While in-person visits may be ideal, often it is more realistic to do some of the check-ins over the phone or to ask a nurse or other practitioner to assist. Often some combination works best. The literature offers little guidance regarding how to taper effectively and even less regarding how providers can monitor outcomes following opioid discontinuation. However, the available data, as well as clinical and ethical sense, favor the need for close contact to improve clinical outcomes.

SHARING SUPPORT

When making medication changes and increasing behavioral strategies, patients can be overwhelmed. Health care providers should allow individuals to communicate their concerns and feelings openly, acknowledging the patient experience and helping to problem-solve and to determine appropriate next steps. This may be a time to adjust goals related to the rate of tapering or activation. However, it may also be sufficient for the patient to be heard, feel validated and understood, and continue with the plan of care.

For patients whose motivation was lacking at treatment initiation, motivational enhancement techniques to boost commitment and reassure support can be helpful. Talking through these challenging times can greatly assist to restore the patient's hope in the process. Some examples of motivational techniques include the following:

- *positive feedback*: "Yes, it did not go exactly as planned, but we can work on that. Let's figure out what got in your way."

- *normalizing experiences*: "It sounds like you overdid it this week, and that made the medication change feel more difficult. Let's talk about how you can avoid a pain flare-up and do what you want this week by pacing."

- *adjusting goals*: "Ups and downs are expected—that is part of life! Please don't be hard on yourself. Let's discuss your goal again and think about a more realistic plan to be successful so you can stay confident. This may be a good time to pause the taper."

- *boosting commitment*: "Do you want to make adjustments to this goal? Let's figure out what we would increase your commitment to accomplishing this. Are there specific obstacles you are concerned about? The good news is you can plan for those and get in the mindset to deal with them as they come."

- *reinforcing effort*: "Starting is always the hardest part. You are taking responsibility for your future, and it will pay off for you. Practicing the skills we've discussed instead of relying on the medications alone is a big deal, and you are doing great. I know you can do this, and I am here for you."

When making changes to opioid medications, the need for close collaboration with each patient and across providers is important; support across providers increases the likelihood of successful deprescribing. When primary care providers don't have enough time to explore patient concerns fully, one of the other practitioners may address patient resistance to the taper recommended by the prescriber. These conversations can be difficult in settings such as primary care, where time is limited to explore patient concerns fully. Health care providers should continue to consider options such as telehealth or telemedicine check-ins and should triage for additional evaluation if indicated. Behavioral health providers may be well poised, given their backgrounds, to share information with other team members. They can assist with consistent messaging and ongoing support for patients who find it challenging to reduce opioids and who need more scaffolding than others to ensure their safety and improve their functioning.

CONCLUSION

Assisting patients at the intersection of pain and opioids is a process that profits from an established rapport and ongoing evaluation. Particularly when individuals are deprescribing, the need for close collaboration is important. A variety of issues can arise when an individual makes changes to medication and lifestyle, and health care providers should feel equipped to address patient concerns and to quell fears. Issues may arise that require adopting a treatment pathway that was not identified previously, such as medication-assisted treatment. However, often the best approach is to address fears and concerns and to make adjustments to the plan of care based on shared decision making. As patients move through the engagement phase, attention shifts to maintaining the progress made during treatment. If gains are made but do not endure, then the patient does not benefit long-term. Maintaining gains is particularly important when reductions have been made to opioid medications, as regression can lead to a decrease in patient safety.

IV PHASE 3: MAINTAINING GAINS

It is the courage to continue that counts.

—Winston Churchill

INTRODUCTION

At this point in treatment, patients have likely improved their functioning, brightened their mood, and decreased their reliance on opioids for pain management. While knowing strategies to positively affect health outcomes is key, practical approaches for sustaining these changes are also essential for long-term improvements (Ory et al., 2010). The focus now shifts to how to maintain gains with a thoughtful appraisal of what works, barriers to effective management, and how to create a realistic framework that sets up individuals for ongoing success. Treatment thus far likely provides ample information regarding typical challenges or vulnerabilities for each person as well as strengths on which to build. The focus of treatment in this phase shifts to strategies for maintaining gains. This phase of treatment is sometimes referred to as *relapse prevention*, and while the term *relapse* has specific associations in the literature on substance use, more broadly it refers to a breakdown or failure to maintain changes in any set of behaviors. Research indicates that some factors are more likely than others to impede the maintenance of changes, for example interpersonal conflicts and negative emotional states (Kwasnicka et al., 2016; Ory et al., 2010). Given that, health care providers should anticipate the potential obstacles and barriers that patients may encounter so that a plan to manage them can be developed and strategies can be practiced during calm times.

One of the most important goals of treatment is to increase self-efficacy regarding pain and opioid management. The longer skills are implemented effectively, the better the chance of long-term success in maintaining that critical sense of personal agency. Expect that individuals with pain will have days, weeks, or even longer periods during which they struggle to implement strategies that they know can be helpful; however, once they have the tools to regain control of their pain experience, they can return to the basics and begin to build again.

Finally, identification of diverse resources to assist patients is a central part of this step. Resources may include other people, such as loved ones or health care professionals; technology-based options, such as online tools or mobile apps; and the ongoing use of therapeutic activities such as yoga, aquatic therapy, or supportive meetings with peers. While maintenance is considered the final phase of treatment, long-term use of integrated approaches should be the goal from initiation. As Stephen Covey (1989) said, "Begin with the end in mind"—to best serve patients, health care providers should weave strategies to get and keep patients engaged with these helpful tools throughout the clinical relationship.

10 DEVELOP A MAINTENANCE PLAN

Maintaining the gains made during the course of treatment is as important as completing the treatment itself. Focusing on maintenance and relapse is recommended (Keefe & Van Horn, 1993): It is not uncommon for individuals with chronic health issues to adopt lifestyle changes while they are in treatment or health-focused programs with good results, only to see symptoms slowly return when the behavior modifications are stopped. This trend has been observed repeatedly in exercise and diet programs (Wu et al., 2009) and highlights the importance of the maintenance phase of treatment. The true measures of success are learning ways to self-manage pain and opioids through various effective strategies and knowing how to seek assistance from others when needed. The goal is to avoid returning to suboptimal pretreatment functioning and opioid use and to feel confident addressing barriers that arise. Once the person acquires a diverse set of skills and strategies to support their pain management and is stable with medication changes, the focus of treatment shifts to maintaining progress and continued growth. In this phase of treatment, health care providers review skills with patients and help to develop a plan to minimize and manage

https://doi.org/10.1037/0000209-011
Chronic Pain and Opioid Management: Strategies for Integrated Treatment,
by J. L. Murphy and S. Rafie

obstacles. Patients should leave treatment confident that the plan will carry them through to continued success.

LESSONS LEARNED

Approaching the end of treatment, health care providers should engage the patient in a review of overall progress toward treatment goals and personal goals, as well as reviewing barriers and facilitators of change. A provider might specifically elicit the patient's subjective report of changes in mood, sleep, energy levels, engagement with valued activities, and social and family participation, as well as their feelings about regaining some self-confidence and sense of identity. The provider might also ask whether they feel more prepared to manage their pain independently, without relying exclusively on opioids. Suggestions for ways to ask individuals to share positive changes they noticed during the course of treatment include the following:

- "Have you become more active?"
- "Has your mood improved?"
- "Are you accomplishing more?"
- "Have you noticed a difference in how you react to your pain?"
- "Do you feel less reliant on opioids for pain management?"
- "Have your loved ones provided any positive feedback about your progress?"

If a patient struggles to identify areas of progress, the provider might share data collected during the initial evaluation regarding mood, sleep, activities, and goals to cue recollection of their starting point, which will likely prompt observations of improved functioning. The health care provider can also share feedback regarding observations of progress over the course of treatment.

Next, the provider can ask the patient to consider factors that supported changes made in treatment as well as obstacles that hindered the process. Facilitators for change may have been identifying a support person or group, scheduling daily activities, or accountability systems, while obstacles may have been elevated pain intensity, low motivation, or psychosocial stress. The provider can also review with the patient how their obstacles were overcome; this review helps to reinforce the active, problem-solving approach used in treatment. These factors will be important considerations in developing a maintenance plan. Table 10.1 includes a list of potential facilitators and obstacles, along with ideas for overcoming challenges.

TABLE 10.1. Factors That Support and Hinder the Process

Facilitators (support the process)	Obstacles (hinder the process)	Ways to overcome obstacles
Scheduled daily activities	Too much unstructured time	Create a weekly calendar Identify regular activities Sign up for a class or volunteer Schedule exercise
Accountability	Lack of accountability	Find an accountability buddy Share goals with others Display short-term goals on the fridge
Managed pain	Elevated pain	Engage in graduated activities Pace activities Divert attention to pleasant activities Practice wellness-focused coping skills
High motivation	Low motivation	Continually remind oneself why these changes are important Place motivational messages in visible places Seek support Start with small goals
Managed stress	Stress at home (e.g., financial, relationship, role conflicts)	Refocus on changeable stressors Set short-term goals Challenge unhelpful thoughts Communicate
Adequate social support	Inadequate social support	Identify alternative sources of support Boost support within existing relationships Seek support groups and activity groups

After identifying areas in which progress was made, it is helpful for the patient and provider to take stock to determine how new skills can and will be used to manage pain and opioids moving forward. Some powerful strategies that can be implemented include the following:

- *understanding*: Increase awareness about the factors that turn up and turn down the volume on pain.

- *reframing*: Check pain-related thoughts regularly to make sure they are helpful and use positive statements to refocus.

- *regulating*: Use relaxation every day to help calm the nervous system and keep the volume down on the pain. Regulation will help a patient to avoid opioid use.

- *pacing*: Plan an approach to all activities to avoid doing too much or too little—a thoughtful approach to everything is key.

- *enjoying*: Pleasant activities create positive emotions and help combat the negative effects of pain and opioids. Make them a priority.

- *preparing*: Use all these skills every day! They will help minimize pain and opioid use increases and will set up a person for a balanced, fulfilling life.

UPDATED GOALS AND A MAINTENANCE PLAN

Looking forward, patients and providers can begin to discuss future directions for progress. Goals for the future that the patient can pursue independently should be discussed as part of the maintenance plan. It is likely that, over the course of treatment, the patient made some progress toward the initial treatment goals while other goals remain unmet. These currently unmet goals are often long-term objectives. This is the time to revisit those goals and objectives to determine updates that need to occur. Unmet goals can be combined with new goals that guide the patient forward; they can be shaped into SMART goals to increase the likelihood of achievement. Examples include the following:

- continue regimented home exercise routine
- increase activities and practice pacing
- increase socialization
- begin hobby
- look for school, work, volunteer possibilities
- maintain daily schedule
- balance activities with relaxation and sleep

After patients have shared their successes and the tools they learned, they should develop a plan for how they will progress toward updated goals while best addressing challenges and potential obstacles. The maintenance plan should integrate skills for pain and opioid management, identify obstacles, anticipate triggers, and provide active strategies to mitigate challenges. Each patient can individualize their plan based on their experience with pain and opioid use and the skills they now have to address concurrent management. While one patient may find that taking a walk has been the best approach to turn down the pain volume, another may feel relaxation has been best to de-stress and helps the person avoid taking another dose of medications.

The four As of successful management can facilitate the patient's reflection as they determine the details of how to minimize and manage pain flare-ups and implement the optimal plan. The health care provider can use the four As to facilitate a conversation with the patient, as follows:

- *Assess* skills: "What are the most effective management skills or strategies you have used? Is there any way to make them more effective?"

- *Avoid* obstacles: "Obstacles are often preventable. Anticipate common challenges you face that would likely turn up the volume on your pain and increase opioid use. What might sidetrack you from using successful management skills? How can you avoid or improve those things?"

- *Anticipate* triggers: "Identify and prepare for triggers—what are they and how will you manage them?"

- *Activate* positive strategies: "You have a lot of excellent tools in your pain and opioid management toolbox now. How can you continue to keep relaxation in your daily life? What pleasant activities will you do for fun and for distraction? What can you do if rethinking pain feels harder than it once did? Name some things you will do to make difficult days better."

Examples of potential pitfalls can be drawn from patients' past experiences, including earlier discussion of how they overcame obstacles during treatment. The purpose of this exercise is to anticipate what may cause a future setback, reinforce problem-solving, and highlight effective strategies to overcome obstacles.

CONTINUED SUPPORT

Patients can maintain a schedule for approaching daily life with a mind toward implementing effective strategies. This schedule may be created with the assistance of a health care provider or may be designed independently by the patient. Regardless, a schedule helps shape the wellness-focused journey and keeps an individual managing pain and opioids on track. Creating a plan that is detailed but also realistic is important. The schedule can be simple but should take into account the following important life activities and events:

- waking time, approximate bedtime
- meals
- physical activities, exercise, stretching

- family time
- pets
- socialization
- religious activities
- hobbies
- work, school, volunteering
- relaxation
- medications

A plan should remind the person what they have accomplished and should support their positive momentum.

As part of ongoing support, providers should continue to be available to the patient. It is important that individuals are reminded that they may contact practitioners if they are stuck and struggling to solve problems independently. Furthermore, they should communicate with health care providers regarding medication issues, such as side effects. If a patient is still in the process of reducing opioids, they should continue with scheduled visits on a regular basis to provide their ongoing input regarding medication changes; this is critical to ensure safety. The plan should integrate skills for managing opioid reductions, especially since patients have experience with tapering and are more familiar with what works best. These options can and should be explored and integrated into the maintenance plan.

The health care provider should offer final thoughts to the person with pain, including reinforcement of messages and encouragement for further progress. Sample statements a provider may use when terminating treatment include the following:

- *remind*: "If you do one of these things you've learned, it will help. If you do them all, it will help a lot."

- *reinforce*: "You've come a long way using these skills and your own motivation to make progress. If you continue using them consistently, you will continue to see progress."

- *prepare*: "There will always be bumps in the road, but you've gotten past them before, and you can do it again. If you stop completely, unwanted symptoms will start to return. If this happens, identify that it is happening and begin using your tools again. It's never too late. The sooner you return to your skills, the easier it will be to get going again."

- *encourage*: "You are strong, and I've seen you dedicate yourself to this. Keep going! You will do great, and great things will come to you!"

This warmth and encouragement from the provider will serve as a final reminder of self-efficacy to the patient. With consistent practice and commitment, they will continue forward.

Clinical Conundrum: Summarizing the Maintenance Plan

Jim has acquired the necessary skills to manage his pain and opioids independently. During this visit, the health care provider focuses on reviewing lessons learned, updated goals, and an action plan based on the four As.

HEALTH CARE PROVIDER (HCP): We have discussed the importance of having a mixed toolbag to manage persistent pain and opioid medications. That means not just relying on pills and rest like the old days but instead using your relaxation techniques, rethinking skills, and activities to feel and function better.

JIM (J): I have to say, there are fewer bad days now. It's not perfect, but the days are overall better than they were.

HCP: That is progress. Remember progress is measured by things like how well you're functioning, what activities you're participating in, and your sleep and mood.

J: Right. The pain is still there, but it's more manageable. I find it doesn't upset me in the same way as it used to now that I have more than opioids to rely on.

HCP: What might sidetrack you from using successful management skills?

J: Probably work getting hectic during crunch season. Realistically, there is no avoiding it, but maybe I can change something with my schedule to be a little more flexible with how I get my hours those weeks.

HCP: That sounds like a good idea. And what are some things you will do to make difficult days better?

J: Most likely relax with some breathing and do some stretching. Try to focus on something I enjoy to take my mind off the pain and not go to meds.

HCP: Perfect. And remember, to keep your mindset in the right direction, it is important to keep practicing these strategies as often as you can. They are already becoming second nature. I am so proud of what you have done for yourself and how much you've improved.

CONCLUSION

Planning is part of succeeding. For a patient to apply their acquired skills consistently on a long-term basis, they must thoughtfully reflect and develop an individualized plan of action. The health care provider can help the patient take stock of their toolbox and focus on what is working well, which increases confidence. Furthermore, the provider can offer reassurance that optimizing pain and opioid management continues to be a team effort and that the patient has the ongoing support of their health care team as well as many other resources. Patients should be encouraged to be open and honest about what complications and obstacles may surface moving forward; patient and provider together can address considerations for how to minimize and manage those challenges.

11 ADDRESS SETBACKS

After an action plan for maintenance has been developed, it is likely that a patient will continue to need options for treatment and support. For behavioral health clinicians, scheduling distinct follow-up sessions may provide the needed scaffolding for long-term success; for other health care professionals, incorporating self-management strategies into regularly scheduled appointments as issues arise may be sufficient. A *booster intervention* is one in which a health care provider assesses a patient's overall functioning since the last contact, their significant life events, and their adherence to the plans set forth regarding management of pain and opioids. It serves as a collaborative contact in which skills are reinforced with the goal of enhancing the patient's confidence in their ability to self-manage their pain and opioids. Some patients may have had setbacks that can be quickly addressed through refresher education and problem-solving. Other patients may have returned to pretreatment functioning levels or may have regressed more significantly; these patients need updated plans for moving forward that are informed by their current status.

https://doi.org/10.1037/0000209-012
Chronic Pain and Opioid Management: Strategies for Integrated Treatment,
by J. L. Murphy and S. Rafie

THE BOOSTER INTERVENTION

During the treatment phase, appointment intervals may be weekly or biweekly and should support the regular acquisition of pain management skills and strategies as well as to support their medication change. Of course, for many disciplines, this frequency is not feasible, and therefore support must be provided when and where it is possible. Regardless, follow-up appointments should be the standard of care to ensure appropriate monitoring, particularly when opioid reductions occur and especially with opioid cessation. This phase is also a time to consider options for support such as telemedicine or telehealth visits that are technology-based, virtual offerings (e.g., web, phone). These support options can serve as complements to in-person visits and can increase support and frequency as needed. When individuals are unable to make it in person or have no emergent issues, these options also offer convenience and enhance accessibility. Discussions, even those that are brief, can be highly valuable.

Assess and Update

This treatment phase might begin with the health care provider obtaining updates regarding the patient's level of functioning since the last appointment. Assessments of activities and mood provide important insight into the patient's functional status in the absence of steady contact with the provider. If the patient experienced significant life events that resulted in distress and impaired functioning, then the provider should pay appropriate attention to addressing these issues by making needed referrals and sharing relevant resources. If the patient reports worsened mood or reduction in activities, the provider should help to identify causal factors and aid in problem-solving and the development of more realistic and adaptive goals.

The focus of the visit should be on assessing the patient's independent pain management and adherence to medication changes. The provider should solicit updates regarding maintenance of skills and strategies learned over the course of treatment, with attention to barriers and facilitators of skill transfer to their home environment. The following conversation starters may facilitate this discussion:

- "Tell me what has been going well over the past few weeks. Thinking back to your mood, sleep, and activities a few months ago, what changes do you notice? What did you do to make that progress?"

- "What hasn't been going so well? What has gotten in your way?"

- "What do you think is helping you move forward?"

- "What is hindering you from making the progress you want?"

- "Which goals do you want to continue? Do you have other goals or ones you would like to change?"

Refresher Education

At this stage, it is likely that the patient is implementing pain self-management strategies independently and is not seeing a health care provider frequently (e.g., weekly). It is likely that the patient would benefit from a brief review of education on chronic pain and opioid management as well as the many factors involved. This review heightens their understanding of why each previously introduced skill is important to continue. The patient's personal story can be used to connect practiced skills to reported progress as well as to other areas that may need improvement. For instance, if they note increased energy and improved mood resulting from increased activities, they may find their sleep improves or their relationships improve. If they have been less active than desired, perhaps an outing has caused an increase in pain and opioid use. These complexities are depicted in Figure 11.1, which can be shared in session to facilitate discussion. The patient may experience improvement in any and all areas, and this improvement can impact other important areas of functioning.

While pain can negatively impact a variety of areas, a shift begins as improvements are made, and people begin to feel better and more like themselves. Changes in mood, due to adaptive thinking or increased activities, may result in improved interpersonal functioning (e.g., communication, intimacy, family participation, socialization), which can then lead to improved physical health factors (e.g., energy level, appetite, sleep) and, ultimately, affect the intensity of the pain. By making improvements in each of the areas shown in Figure 11.1, the person begins to manage their pain and opioids better. Revisiting this basic pain education serves multiple purposes:

- understanding that use of skills leads to improved functioning
- reinforcing that a diverse set of skills and tools to manage pain reduces dependence on opioids as the primary method of pain management
- instilling hope that continued effort will result in further progress

People cope with pain in various ways, which can be roughly divided into two categories: wellness-focused coping and illness-focused coping

FIGURE 11.1. Factors Involved in the Pain Experience

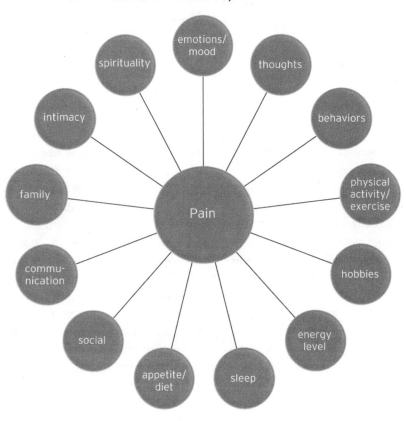

Table 11.1). These terms were originally coined by Jensen et al. (1995) to distinguish the strategies that promote functioning and wellness from those that further illness.

Wellness-focused coping strategies help patients improve functionality. They should be applied regularly and consistently. In a broad sense, patients will want to maintain a daily schedule of activities, including graduated activity, socialization, and relaxation. Specific skills that are important to continue include staying active, pleasant activity scheduling, reframing negative or unhelpful thoughts, and dedicating time to relaxation exercises, such as diaphragmatic breathing or autogenic relaxation. When combined, these skills help to manage stress and reactions and to prevent flare-ups. Activity pacing should be used not only to begin and increase certain physical activities but also to sustain activity levels throughout a week or day. This pacing is particularly useful for moderating activities as medications

TABLE 11.1. Illness-Focused Coping Contrasted With Wellness-Focused Coping

Illness-focused coping	Wellness-focused coping
Resting, guarding	Deep breathing
Taking more opioids than prescribed	Taking nonopioid analgesic medication
Asking for help	Going for a walk or stretching
Avoiding seeing anyone	Calling a friend
Thinking the worst	Challenging unhelpful thoughts
Extending time off or down time	Setting a goal for the day
Overdoing activities	Pacing your activities
Stressing about past, worrying about future	Meditating or praying
Focusing on the pain	Reading or playing a game
Relying on medication alone	Trying a physical therapy tool, such as self-massage or foam rolling

changes become stabilized. Finally, managing pain flare-ups optimally requires using a combination of the previously described skills and strategies as well as continuing medications as prescribed.

Illness-focused coping strategies, which include resting and isolating, may help momentarily but can hinder long term functioning. Illness-focused coping often contradicts the goals of wellness-focused coping, which focuses on proactive pain self-management. The use of illness-focused coping strategies should be minimized. Patients benefit from reviewing the importance of pacing activities, rather than overdoing or avoiding them altogether. A key point for a provider to reinforce is the consequences of patients adjusting their own medications based on activities or pain intensity, particularly when they take more than the amount prescribed. Self-medication can result in the patient running out of medications early and can be dangerous to their health. The provider should consider the ongoing challenges for the person in pain and approach the conversation with empathy, while redirecting them to their alternative pain management tools when they feel the urge to take more medications.

Jumping Over Hurdles

Together with the patient, the health care provider should identify and address the obstacles that occurred since the last visit. Most commonly, an obstacle is loss of motivation after the support of and accountability to the provider was removed. However, there are many reasons that a person with chronic pain can experience a setback as they move forward independently. Increases in pain may have resulted in reduction in activities and a gradual loss of motivation and forward momentum. Other common issues are increased negative thoughts, family stress, and worries regarding work, finances, or the future. To help the patient problem-solve, a provider might suggest the following steps:

1. *Explore and analyze*: Think through the situation as an observer to identify where the plan went off course.
2. *Define the problem*: Clearly identify the issue perpetuating reduced functioning.
3. *Brainstorm solutions*: Consider any and all possible solutions.
4. *Narrow down*: Identify the most realistic and effective solution.
5. *Action plan*: Integrate the solution into a modified action plan.
6. *Evaluate outcomes*: Determine whether the solution was effective, and decide how to adjust the plan if the issue is not fully resolved.

The last step may be accomplished outside of treatment or perhaps during another booster session.

The goal of treatment always centers on bolstering the patient's independence and confidence in self-management of their pain and medications. Handouts and worksheets can be useful tools to aid their ongoing wellness journey. Handouts specific to the identified obstacles, as well as those containing general tips and encouragement, are useful. For example, if a patient's problem is related to frequent bouts of irritability and anger, a handout describing anger management skills is appropriate. Handouts that are generally useful to provide during the booster session include the following:

- tips on managing pain flare-ups
- what to expect when tapering opioids
- a note of encouragement from the health care provider
- stress management skills
- anger management skills
- coping self-statements

Handouts on these topics can be created by the health care provider or easily found on the internet.

How skills will be integrated into individuals' lives should also be discussed, regardless of whether further follow-up is planned. This conversation may include discussion of relaxation or mindfulness practice, development of an activity schedule, daily journaling, or community-based support groups. Considerations for home practice are based on areas of need. If the person reported struggling to maintain a regular independent exercise plan because they lack an activity buddy, then they could be encouraged to search for a local walking group or a local peer support group for people with chronic pain.

Clinical Conundrum: Dealing With Setbacks

Jim reveals that after a spell of bronchitis, he did not return to his usual activities. In fact, he started taking more days off work after realizing he was taking more pills to get through the day and was not active outside of work. He continued with his relaxation exercises and maintained a balanced attitude, but he was aware of the setback. The health care provider assists Jim in analyzing the situation, problem-solving, and developing an action plan.

HEALTH CARE PROVIDER (HCP): Where do you think things went off course with your activities?

JIM (J): Well, once I was feeling better, I should have started back up again with the stretching and maybe even some other activities, but I just got comfortable with not doing those things.

HCP: I get it. Doing those helpful things becomes a habit, but so does not doing those things. Let's talk about some possible solutions. What might be helpful to get you going again?

J: I should probably tell my wife that I need to do it, so she can remind me. Or we can even do the stretches or go for a walk together.

HCP: Those are great ideas. Any other potential solutions?

J: I could sign up for some of the classes at my gym and commit to a schedule. I have been wanting to do that.

HCP: For now, which would you say is the more realistic solution, the one you feel most confident about?

J: Probably getting my wife on board to do a 30-minute stretch break together every day.

HCP: Alright. So what steps are needed to accomplish this solution?

J: I'll talk to her when I get home and come up with a plan for what time of day is best and what we'll do. I already have the exercises that I was doing from physical therapy, so that part is easy.

HCP: Perfect. We can plan to check in to see how that plan worked out.

More Booster Interventions

The patient and health care provider decide together on the appropriate plan for follow-up. Depending on the severity of setbacks or the person's ability to return to their skills easily, more extensive support and appointments may be necessary. If the patient reports minimal challenges or is able to return to more adaptive pain management skills easily, then treatment needs may be limited. The provider should always reinforce individuals' personal strengths, emphasize positive decisions that have been made, encourage the patient to identify their own progress, and reflect on their ability to grow and create change based on their choices. This affirmation of self-efficacy supports their continued work on their wellness journey.

BACK TO BASELINE

Regardless of how prepared patients feel for independence, they are dealing with a chronic condition, and some will return to something resembling pre-morbid functioning. This could mean reengaging in an unhelpful pattern of fear and avoidance, using or increasing opioid analgesics, or withdrawing from friends and family. This scenario presents challenges for both patient and provider and is important to carefully assess and address to determine a plan for moving forward and to better prepare for future obstacles.

Relapse or Setback?

There is a significant difference between a relapse and a setback. *Setbacks* are temporary lapses in progress, whereas a *relapse* is prolonged and happens when a person stops maintaining their goals and returns to baseline functioning. A setback can be thought of as a road closure or bump in the road, whereas a relapse is coming to a screeching halt and giving up to go home. In this analogy, one slows down for a bump in the road, then continues forward. Both are expected along the road of functional rehabilitation and medication reduction. The key is to recognize that an event has occurred, gauge the severity, and respond appropriately.

Treatment approaches differ for setbacks and relapse. If a road closure was anticipated in advance, perhaps one looks for an alternate route; however, often the closure is abrupt. If the person is at the point where they give up and go home, then the response should include uncovering why they left the house in the first place to determine the best route to the destination. It is expected that patients will experience life stressors, pain, and other personal challenges that may cause a lapse in goal-directed behavior. This lapse may start as a temporary setback, but if the person never corrects the course, then the setback becomes a relapse.

Relapses have many different causes, including problems at work, interpersonal difficulties, economic problems, ongoing emotional or psychiatric issues, and pain flare-ups. The following signs indicate a relapse:

- increased stress or emotional crisis
- loss of interest in being active or engaging in hobbies
- changes in behavior
- taking more medications than prescribed
- isolating or withdrawing
- emergency room visits

Severity of relapse is indicated by the number of signs the person is demonstrating as well as the time since the relapse started. The response should be tailored based on the severity of the relapse and specific domains affected. Motivational enhancement techniques are useful when a health care provider engages a patient in this discussion. Strategies and suggestions to drive the conversation include the following:

- *identify triggers*: "What was happening around the time that you stopped your usual activities or started taking more medication?"
- *identify emotions*: "How were you feeling at that time?"
- *identify thoughts*: "Can you identify any thoughts that led to your decision to go back to your old prescription?"
- *adapt*: "Having looked at this situation more closely, is there anything you would do differently in the future to prevent this from happening?"

Emotional Reactions

It is unrealistic to assume that growth and progress will be continuous. Bumps in the road are expected and are not signs of failure on the part of the patient or the health care practitioner, whereas a relapse can be more challenging for both. Provider and patient may have automatic thoughts and reactions to the relapse. Exploration of these reactions may provide insight that is useful, especially for the patient, and can be incorporated into the discussion. Table 11.2 lists common emotional reactions to relapse.

The patient is likely to have a myriad of feelings surrounding this regression. Guilt is common and is associated with a sense of failing to achieve goals and disappointing others. Shame may follow, focused more on shortcomings or personal defects. The person may experience thoughts

TABLE 11.2. Common Emotional Reactions to Relapse

Patient reactions	Provider reactions	Motivating response
Failure	Failure	"Relapse is a common challenge."
Guilt	Inadequacy	"You are doing your best."
Shame	Frustration	"You deserve credit for recognizing the issue before it went on any longer."
Self-blame	Blaming	"Let's see what we can learn from this."
Helplessness	Helplessness	"You've had a lot of successes before this, and you will again."
Hopelessness	Hopelessness	"It's about progress, not perfection."

of self-blame and negative self-judgments. And, finally, the patient may feel disheartened that their efforts thus far seem to have been for naught and may return to feelings of helplessness or hopelessness. The provider may have similar feelings of failure and inadequacy, viewing the relapse as a failure on their part as a health care provider. They may also experience feelings of frustration, resulting from attempts to place blame or potential perceptions or misperceptions of patient resistance or refusal to cooperate. Like the patient, the provider may feel a sense of helplessness or hopelessness that they cannot affect the outcome and that nothing will change.

Despite one's own reactions, it is important for a provider to remain nonjudgmental and to avoid shaming individuals who relapse. Remaining supportive is especially important given that the patient is likely to be experiencing negative emotions about their relapse. When the provider continues to provide a safe treatment environment that is focused on problem-solving, the patient will return to work through these challenges.

Reframing Relapse

One way providers can help patients who have relapsed is to reframe relapse so that it is not seen as failure. Progress is not a steady course of forward movement. In fact, temporary slowing and occasional backward movement is normal and expected. In the face of these challenges, growth occurs. Patients learn more about their own patterns, and they become better prepared to deal with future detours. There is no failure, only opportunities to learn and do better next time. It is natural for both patient and provider to be disappointed in unrealized treatment objectives; however, in any rehabilitation or recovery treatment, setbacks and relapses are expected. They are realities and should be reviewed throughout the treatment process. This normalization enhances the patient's willingness to share openly and address the problem, continuing forward rather than being stricken by guilt or shame.

Ambivalence

Exploration of the patient's thoughts and feelings regarding their relapse may lead to discovery of ambivalence about their intentions in treatment. The patient may lose motivation and may regress to the precontemplation or contemplation stages of change; it is also possible they never advanced beyond these stages. As such, an important focus of this discussion is to elicit self-motivating statements that will increase the patient's self-responsibility and boost self-esteem. The following questions provide helpful examples:

- "Let's look at the positive side of where you are right now. Tell me, what do you like about taking oxycodone at the higher dose?"

- "Now, let's look at the other side. What about the higher dose do you dislike? What are your concerns about returning to a higher dose?"

- "What led you to the decision that perhaps you need to make a change in your medications?"

- "It sounds as if you might be better off continuing with your original medications, as you were before. Why make a change at all?"

- "What other factors do you think might be playing a part in the challenges you're having right now?"

- "It seems more important to you to stay on the higher dose than to continue the plan of taking a balanced pain management approach. It does take a lot of motivation to see the plan through, and I'm not sure you are there. Do you think we should move forward or go back to the original prescription?"

These questions may elicit statements that move the patient toward their original health goals. They may be struggling to come up with any concerns about staying with their original prescription or giving up their active pain management strategies. Ideally, the patient cultivates their own motivation; however, the provider's responses can foster this motivation.

Responding

The health care provider should always maintain a flexible and non-judgmental approach in treatment. Even when the patient is struggling to identify their own motivation, the provider should allow adequate space for the person to process their own thoughts. The clinician can and should listen actively, with empathy and compassion for the struggle. The following clinical skills and responses can be very powerful tools in aiding the patient's contemplation:

- *remain nonjudgmental*: "What concerns you about your current pattern?"

- *listen actively*: "Sounds like you're still deciding what's best for you."

- *empathize*: "I can see why you would be concerned."

- *reflect*: "It's hard for you to see yourself feeling this way long-term."

- *summarize*: "On the one hand, cutting back the medications would offer you more freedom to focus on your health. On the other hand, going back to your original dose may get you out of feeling the way you do right now."

In essence, providers should limit advice-giving and suggestions in favor of listening to the patient and helping them sort out their true desires.

Adapting

Many different strategies for managing a relapse can be discussed, either during the initial treatment phase or in response to a relapse. The best course of action is for a provider to help the patient prepare for potential issues that can arise. Figure 11.2 lists a set of strategies that can be used to respond to a relapse. These strategies can be shared with the patient at any point in

FIGURE 11.2. Strategies for Responding to Setbacks and Relapse

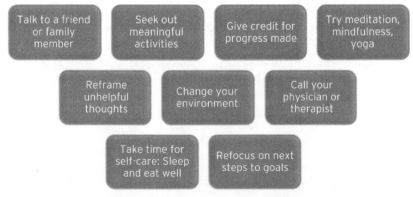

treatment that seems appropriate or during a follow-up visit if a relapse has occurred. Some can be applied by the patient without outside involvement, while others require the support of key members of their support team. Most of the strategies do not depend on the provider facilitating independent problem-solving. If another treatment intervention is indicated, the provider and patient may need to discuss how to contact or consult with other health care providers to assist. Despite any problems with implementation, if patients consistently use the strategies, the acquired skills will become more automatic and lead to improved outcomes. A diverse approach is always going to return the best results; thus, patients are encouraged to start with one or more of these strategies and incorporate their own approaches that work.

Clinical Conundrum: Addressing Relapse

During treatment, Jim reduced his daily dose of opioids and learned to manage his pain independently. Jim contacts his provider to request a follow-up visit to discuss problems with his pain management. He states he has been sleeping late regularly and is having a hard time getting to work in the morning. At work, he avoids the more physical work and is only doing enough to get by. He discloses that recently his mood has been worse, and he is back to not seeing friends because of his fatigue. Eventually, he reveals he started taking more than his currently prescribed opioids by adding doses from an old prescription he still had. He is unsure if he wants to continue with the tapering plan. The health care provider remains nonjudgmental while identifying antecedents to the relapse as a means to determine next steps.

HEALTH CARE PROVIDER (HCP): What was happening around the time that you stopped your usual activities and started taking more medication?

JIM (J): It was after a while of feeling more depressed. I don't even know why exactly. I just started lying around more. I thought a lot about what we talked about, but I couldn't get going.

HCP: Sounds like you're still deciding what's best for you. Can you identify any thoughts that led to your decision to go back to your old prescription?

J: Sometimes I think all the effort to push myself to deal with the pain just isn't worth the effort and it's easier to just take the pill. I know that sounds bad. I'm just being honest.

HCP: I can see why you would be having a hard time with this decision. It seems like increasing your opioids may get you out of feeling the way you do right now. Given your history with medication and the lack of improvement in your life, we need to examine that carefully. But first, is there anything you would do differently in the future to prevent this type of setback from happening again?

J: I probably could have caught it sooner and made an appointment with you. My wife was saying it, too. Next time I see myself starting to want to stay home all the time, I'll make an appointment before things go too far.

HCP: That's a great idea. The sooner we can talk about things, the sooner we can get a plan together to help you feel better.

J: And maybe I can bring my wife with me next time. That way, she can learn some ways to help get me back on track when I'm in that down place. I think that would help.

HCP: Or even better, before you get there. This happens to many people dealing with pain—there are ups and downs. The important thing is that you're learning more about yourself so you can be healthier and respond to situations mindfully.

CONCLUSION

The phases of treatment are fluid; they reflect the realities of life. Both patients and providers should understand that, like chronic health conditions, treatment trajectories have ups and downs. Difficult moments or phases are expected during pain and opioid management, so preparing for what to do when they occur is critical. Setbacks and relapses should be handled by marrying compassion with active strategies for addressing concerns. Part of this process is ensuring that individuals have sufficient resources to assist them with optimally managing the intersection of pain and opioids.

12 REINFORCE RESOURCES

Reducing opioids and using a set of skills and strategies for effective pain management is a lifelong process. Health care professionals have an important role to provide information and resources to patients for self-management of their health. Many resources assist with ongoing self-management of pain and opioids, from support organizations to peer support groups. This chapter includes a review of resources, along with ideas for further exploration.

SUPPORT ORGANIZATIONS AND PEER SUPPORT

Many major organizations provide information that is helpful and hopeful to people managing pain and opioids. These organizations provide unique platforms to bring together people with a common goal of living better despite pain, whether they are in the same geographic area or scattered across the globe. Disorder-specific organizations focus on temporomandibular joint disease, complex regional pain syndrome, migraines, endometriosis,

https://doi.org/10.1037/0000209-013
Chronic Pain and Opioid Management: Strategies for Integrated Treatment,
by J. L. Murphy and S. Rafie

and others. Organizations often provide educational content for people with pain who use opioids and their loved ones, and they create avenues for peer support group formation. Some of these groups may be formed locally; others can be held virtually to expand to a broader reach. Organizations have trained group facilitators who hold meetings across the country. Organizations may also provide resources that benefit providers who are seeking education related to pain, opioids, substance use, and medication safety, which may also help address concerns voiced by prescribers (Martino et al., 2020).

Organizations with resources and support for people with chronic pain include the following:

- American Chronic Pain Association (https://www.theacpa.org/)
- U.S. Pain Foundation (https://uspainfoundation.org/)
- Pain Connection (https://painconnection.org/)
- Reflex Sympathetic Dystrophy Syndrome Association (https://rsds.org/)
- For Grace (http://www.forgrace.org/)
- Chronic Pain Self-Management Program (https://www.selfmanagement resource.com/programs/small-group/chronic-pain-self-management/)
- My Migraine Team (https://www.mymigraineteam.com/)

Organizations with resources and support for people struggling with opioids include the following:

- Substance Abuse and Mental Health Services Administration (https://www.samhsa.gov/ or 1-800-662-HELP)
- Shatterproof: Stronger than Addiction (https://www.shatterproof.org/)
- SMART Recovery: Self-Management and Recovery Training (https://www.smartrecovery.org/)
- National Institute on Drug Abuse (https://www.drugabuse.gov/)
- Prescribe to Prevent (https://prescribetoprevent.org/)

LOCAL ACTIVITY GROUPS AND CLASSES

Local groups can be a source of building a great support network within the community that focuses on self-management of health goals. Groups may be formed through mutual acquaintances, mutual health conditions, or common interests. Individuals who seek additional motivation or account-ability for maintaining physical activities may find that walking groups or exercise classes provide necessary structure and the opportunity for social-ization. Individuals seeking increased social connection may find groups that meet to participate in shared interests and hobbies, such as crafting or fishing. Adaptive activity groups, which modify or adapt activities depending on the needs of participants, can also be found. Local activity groups and classes that are commonly available include the following:

- gyms and YMCA
- walking groups found online (e.g., https://www.meetup.com/)
- hobby groups found from community advertising (e.g., at crafts stores or sports stores)
- recreational classes found through the library
- social groups found in the newspaper
- spiritual groups

SUPPORT FROM LOVED ONES

An important area for providers to discuss with patients is support from close relationships, such as a spouse, partner, sibling, parent, or friend. The people dearest to the patient hold great potential to provide consistent support throughout the journey with pain and opioids. However, relationships may have become strained if the patient has a history of poor coping and maladaptive behaviors, and family systems can become highly complicated when pain and opioids are involved. Loved ones can be both helpful and harmful, the latter occurring often without intent. For support to be effective, loved ones must understand what chronic pain is and is not, the role of opioids in pain management, reasonable expectations for treatments, and how to support the patient in a way that is therapeutic. Loved ones can also play an important role in helping patients remain accountable and on track toward their goals. Thus, social support can and should be an integral part of the treatment and maintenance plan.

The following strategies are effective ways for health care providers to help patients enhance social support:

- Identify how relationships may have been affected by past coping behaviors identify elements of healthy relationships.

- Provide educational materials to the patient regarding chronic pain and opioids that can also be shared with family.

- Encourage patients to share what they learn in treatment with close family and friends who also need to learn more about pain, opioids, and expectations for treatment outcomes.

- Discuss how close friends or family members can help with accountability for taking medications as prescribed and maintaining use of active pain-management skills.

- Discuss ways in which loved ones may intend to help but work against patients' personal goals.

- Encourage an identified support person to attend a booster visit.

PSYCHOLOGICAL SUPPORT AND COUNSELING

Over the course of treatment, it may become apparent to the health care provider that other factors are involved in the patient's overall functioning. As has been discussed at length, multimorbidities are commonplace within this population. Psychiatric issues such as posttraumatic stress disorder and substance use disorders all closely interact with functioning and progress, as do issues such as insomnia. It is important that providers address comorbidities appropriately, including an evaluation for acuity level to determine treatment needs.

The following strategies may be used by providers to help patients find psychological support and improve their mental health:

- Recommend relevant self-help resources.

- Provide the National Crisis Hotline number so that patients can reach out for additional support any time by calling 1-800-273-TALK (8255).

- Consider recommending a 12-step program for individuals who are considering initiating or maintaining abstinence from alcohol or other drugs.

- Refer patients to a pain psychology therapist to address comorbid chronic pain, insomnia, and mood symptoms.

- Refer patients to a primary care or general mental health provider for outpatient psychotherapy to address posttraumatic stress disorder or mild-to-moderate mood disorders.

- Consider referring patients to a psychiatrist for medication management.

- Suggest secondary-level, intensive outpatient programs for co-occurring disorders, substance use disorders, and moderate-to-severe mood disorders.

- Engage tertiary-level, psychiatric or medical inpatient hospitalization for acute crises.

TECH TOOLS

Technology provides a vast number of tools that can be useful for maintaining progress both during and after treatment, many of which are no cost or low cost. The opportunity to reach support via the internet and utilize health-focused applications enhances the person's ability to self-manage their pain and opioids. Given that technology is ever-changing and continuously evolving, the resources shared here are general and should guide health care providers to appropriate tools to recommend to patients. Technology tools and resources include the following:

- audio and video recordings and smart device applications to guide relaxation practice
- fitness trackers to monitor physical activity
- smart pill boxes that track adherence to prescribed medication regimens
- online support groups
- motivational videos that inspire mind over matter, perseverance, and personal growth
- virtual reality platforms to assist with relaxation, physical engagement, and education
- smart device applications for tracking activities, exercise, mood, and other health goals
- alarms as daily reminders for regular movement, relaxation, and other goals
- medication alarms to stay on schedule, if prescribed to take opioids on a schedule
- forums for communicating directly with other people with pain

CONCLUSION

The most effective outcomes often come from using a multifaceted approach that combines all of the pieces we have available into the best puzzle we can create. Fortunately, abundant resources are available help patients maximize their use of integrated strategies for pain and opioid management. Technology-based options, such as applications that can be used anywhere to encourage the use of relaxation techniques and activity engagement, have proved to be especially helpful. In addition, loved ones and peers are key in recovery and rehabilitation; their involvement should be encouraged. Patients and health care providers should work together to evaluate what is needed to optimize the chances for success.

Afterword: Conclusions

The relationship between chronic pain and the use of opioid analgesics is a long and complicated one. The United States has struggled with opioid-related issues in a cyclic fashion since the 1800s, vacillating between lax and limited prescribing practices. Amidst the fallout of the current opioid crisis, one favorable outcome is an increased interest in nonpharmacological treatments for pain. While legislators, policymakers, and guideline writers have indicated that multidisciplinary care addressing the biopsychosocial factors relevant in pain experiences and outcomes is recommended (Dowell et al., 2016; Institute of Medicine, 2011; U.S. Department of Health and Human Services, 2019b; U.S. Department of Veterans Affairs and Department of Defense, 2017; U.S. Office of the Assistant Secretary for Health, 2016), many patients and even many health care providers have yet to shift their biomedically focused mindset. The crux of the issue lies in the long-standing conceptualization of all pain in acute terms—as a symptom to be cured rather than as an ongoing condition requiring multifaceted management. This myopic conceptualization falls short for the millions of Americans dealing with chronic pain every day. A result of this belief is that many people possess the false understanding that chronic pain can be eradicated if only the "right" intervention is found, discovered, shared with them—that a deus ex machina will somehow save us from this suffering.

This, in part, led to an overreliance on opioids for so many people, although a variety of other important factors contributed to this perfect storm. In the late 1990s, consensus statements from prominent pain-focused

https://doi.org/10.1037/0000209-014
Chronic Pain and Opioid Management: Strategies for Integrated Treatment,
by J. L. Murphy and S. Rafie

professional societies, direct input from patients to treat pain more effectively, and aggressive marketing of a new drug called Oxycontin to primary care providers (Rummans et al., 2018) all contributed to and culminated in a dramatic increase in opioid prescribing. Specifically, the annual number of prescriptions for Oxycontin, a long-acting extended-release medication intended for individuals with chronic pain, increased from 670,000 to 6.2 million between 1997 and 2002; during that same period, the total number of opioids prescribed increased by 45 million (Rummans et al., 2018). This combination suggested that opioids were T-H-E answer for those who were desperately seeking one. These potent medications were shared more liberally than they should have been and were used as a unidimensional panacea for pain. As recently as 2017, a National Survey on Drug Use and Health indicated that 11.1 million people aged 12 and older self-reported that they had misused prescription pain relievers in the past year, which is likely an underestimate (Center for Behavioral Health Statistics and Quality, 2018). Moreover, data indicate that approximately 1 of every 10 people over 12 years old will develop opioid use disorder (OUD), with only about one fourth of them receiving treatment (Center for Behavioral Health Statistics and Quality, 2018).

The reality is that while analgesics—preferably those that are prescribed judiciously and with a thorough risk–benefit analysis—are an important part of a comprehensive pain treatment plan, they must not be the entire plan. It is unreasonable to expect that people can achieve optimal functioning through a single approach. A full range of treatments must be engaged, including behavioral health strategies that hold an evidence base for treating both pain and substance use, such as cognitive behavioral therapy (CBT). Undeniably, there is a significant need for research and clinical guidance for integrated approaches to pain and opioid use. On a positive note, various funded trials are in progress (Darnall et al., 2019; Sandhu et al., 2019; Vowles et al., 2019), and recent research suggests that approaches such as CBT can help with both pain and opioid management (Garland et al., 2020). Any information gleaned from emerging research will help practitioners increase understanding, improve treatment, and provide consistent messaging to this population.

While we have seen changes in policy regarding increased restrictions on opioids, we have not seen commensurate increases in the availability of comprehensive pain management. This discrepancy is both unjust and unethical to those who suffer from chronic pain and is related to two separate but potentially related issues. First, guidelines and data suggest that patients should engage in a variety of treatments that are not currently covered by insurance and are not broadly available. Reimbursement for comprehensive pain management to include nonpharmacological options such as behavioral pain medicine, much of which has more and higher quality evidence than the medical/pharmacological options, should be covered by payers. This coverage is needed to adequately address the co-occurring crises involving pain and opioids. Second, there is an increased need for training and education in behavioral pain medicine strategies (Darnall et al., 2016) so that access to evidence-based treatments such as CBT are more widely available. Funding should be provided to assist states in educating their health care providers to better assist individuals with pain, including those who are also using opioids in an attempt to quell their pain. In addition, training across disciplines should be prioritized so that practitioners in specialties such as pain medicine have a better understanding of OUD. These conditions do not exist in silos and should not be treated as such.

The biggest challenge is how to shift the zeitgeist—to move the populace from pointing fingers outward for someone else to "fix" their health-related issues and instead encourage individuals to become formidable agents of change in their own health care. As a society, we must shift the focus to maximizing overall wellness, which incorporates the many facets of the whole person and the importance of behavioral choices. When we help arm individuals with tools to improve their capacity to manage pain and opioids, they are empowered not just to achieve improved health but to live life more fully.

References

Abbott, A. D., Tyni-Lenné, R., & Hedlund, R. (2011). Leg pain and psychological variables predict outcome 2–3 years after lumbar fusion surgery. *European Spine Journal*, *20*(10), 1626–1634. https://doi.org/10.1007/s00586-011-1709-6

Afari, N., Ahumada, S. M., Wright, L. J., Mostoufi, S., Golnari, G., Reis, V., & Cuneo, J. G. (2014). Psychological trauma and functional somatic syndromes: A systematic review and meta-analysis. *Psychosomatic Medicine*, *76*(1), 2–11. https://doi.org/10.1097/PSY.0000000000000010

Ajo, R., Segura, A., Inda, M.-D.-M., Margarit, C., Ballester, P., Martínez, E., Ferrández, G., Sánchez-Barbie, Á., & Peiró, A. M. (2017). Erectile dysfunction in patients with chronic pain treated with opioids. *Medicina Clínica*, *149*(2), 49–54. https://doi.org/10.1016/j.medcli.2016.12.038

Ajo, R., Segura, A., Inda, M. M., Planelles, B., Martínez, L., Ferrández, G., Sánchez, A., Margarit, C., & Peiró, A.-M. (2016). Opioids increase sexual dysfunction in patients with non-cancer pain. *Journal of Sexual Medicine*, *13*(9), 1377–1386. https://doi.org/10.1016/j.jsxm.2016.07.003

Alperstein, D., & Sharpe, L. (2016). The efficacy of motivational interviewing in adults with chronic pain: A meta-analysis and systematic review. *The Journal of Pain*, *17*(4), 393–403. https://doi.org/10.1016/j.jpain.2015.10.021

American Psychiatric Association. (2013). *Diagnostic and statistical manual of mental disorders* (5th ed.). https://doi.org/10.1176/appi.books.9780890425596

Ang, D. C., Kaleth, A. S., Bigatti, S., Mazzuca, S. A., Jensen, M. P., Hilligoss, J., Slaven, J., & Saha, C. (2013). Research to encourage exercise for fibromyalgia (REEF): Use of motivational interviewing, outcomes from a randomized-controlled trial. *The Clinical Journal of Pain*, *29*(4), 296–304. https://doi.org/10.1097/AJP.0b013e318254ac76

Angelou, M. (1994, November 2). *What would you save in a fire* [Television interview]? The Oprah Winfrey Show. http://www.oprah.com/oprahs-lifeclass/the-powerful-lesson-maya-angelou-taught-oprah-video

Arntz, A., Dreessen, L., & De Jong, P. (1994). The influence of anxiety on pain: Attentional and attributional mediators. *Pain, 56*(3), 307–314. https://doi.org/10.1016/0304-3959(94)90169-4

Arteta, J., Cobos, B., Hu, Y., Jordan, K., & Howard, K. (2016). Evaluation of how depression and anxiety mediate the relationship between pain catastrophizing and prescription opioid misuse in a chronic pain population. *Pain Medicine, 17*(2), 295–303.

Asmundson, G. J. G., & Katz, J. (2009). Understanding the co-occurrence of anxiety disorders and chronic pain: State-of-the-art. *Depression and Anxiety, 26*(10), 888–901. https://doi.org/10.1002/da.20600

Bair, M. J., Matthias, M. S., Nyland, K. A., Huffman, M. A., Stubbs, D. L., Kroenke, K., & Damush, T. M. (2009). Barriers and facilitators to chronic pain self-management: A qualitative study of primary care patients with comorbid musculoskeletal pain and depression. *Pain Medicine, 10*(7), 1280–1290. https://doi.org/10.1111/j.1526-4637.2009.00707.x

Bair, M. J., Robinson, R. L., Katon, W., & Kroenke, K. (2003). Depression and pain comorbidity: A literature review. *Archives of Internal Medicine, 163*(20), 2433–2445. https://doi.org/10.1001/archinte.163.20.2433

Baldini, A., Von Korff, M., & Lin, E. H. B. (2012). A review of potential adverse effects of long-term opioid therapy: A practitioner's guide. *The Primary Care Companion for CNS Disorders, 14*(3). https://doi.org/10.4088/PCC.11m01326

Bandura, A. (1977). Self-efficacy: Toward a unifying theory of behavioral change. *Psychological Review, 84*(2), 191–215. https://doi.org/10.1037/0033-295X.84.2.191

Bandura, A. (1982). Self-efficacy mechanism in human agency. *American Psychologist, 37*(2), 122–147. https://doi.org/10.1037/0003-066X.37.2.122

Banta-Green, C. J., Von Korff, M., Sullivan, M. D., Merrill, J. O., Doyle, S. R., & Saunders, K. (2010). The prescribed opioids difficulties scale: A patient-centered assessment of problems and concerns. *The Clinical Journal of Pain, 26*(6), 489–497. https://doi.org/10.1097/AJP.0b013e3181e103d9

Barry, D. T., Beitel, M., Cutter, C. J., Fiellin, D. A., Kerns, R. D., Moore, B. A., Oberleitner, L., Madden, L. M., Liong, C., Ginn, J., & Schottenfeld, R. S. (2019). An evaluation of the feasibility, acceptability, and preliminary efficacy of cognitive-behavioral therapy for opioid use disorder and chronic pain. *Drug and Alcohol Dependence, 194*, 460–467. https://doi.org/10.1016/j.drugalcdep.2018.10.015

Bawa, F. L. M., Mercer, S. W., Atherton, R. J., Clague, F., Keen, A., Scott, N. W., & Bond, C. M. (2015). Does mindfulness improve outcomes in patients with chronic pain? Systematic review and meta-analysis. *British Journal of General Practice, 65*(635), e387–e400. https://doi.org/10.3399/bjgp15X685297

Beasley, M. J., Ferguson-Jones, E. A., & Macfarlane, G. J. (2017). Treatment expectations but not preference affect outcome in a trial of CBT and exercise for pain. *Canadian Journal of Pain (Revue Canadienne De La Douleur)*, *1*(1), 161–170. https://doi.org/10.1080/24740527.2017.1384297

Beck, A. T. (1964). Thinking and depression: Theory and therapy. *Archives of General Psychiatry*, *10*, 561–571. https://doi.org/10.1001/archpsyc. 1964.01720240015003

Beck, A. T. (2008). The evolution of the cognitive model of depression and its neurobiological correlates. *The American Journal of Psychiatry*, *165*, 969–977. https://doi.org/10.1176/appi.ajp.2008.08050721

Beck, A. T., Epstein, N., Brown, G., & Steer, R. A. (1988). An inventory for measuring clinical anxiety: Psychometric properties. *Journal of Consulting and Clinical Psychology*, *56*(6), 893–897. https://doi.org/10.1037/0022-006X.56.6.893

Beck, A. T., Rush, A. J., Shaw, B. F., & Emery, G. (1979). *Cognitive therapy of depression*. Guilford Press.

Beck, A. T., Steer, R. A., & Brown, G. K. (1996). *Manual for the Beck Depression Inventory–II*. Psychological Corporation.

Beck, J. S. (2005). *Cognitive therapy for challenging problems*. Guilford Press.

Bee, P., McBeth, J., MacFarlane, G. J., & Lovell, K. (2016). Managing chronic widespread pain in primary care: A qualitative study of patient perspectives and implications for treatment delivery. *BMC Musculoskeletal Disorders*, *17*, Article 354. https://doi.org/10.1186/s12891-016-1194-5

Benson, H., Beary, J. F., & Carol, M. P. (1974). The relaxation response. *Psychiatry*, *37*(1), 37–46. https://doi.org/10.1080/00332747.1974.11023785

Berna, C., Kulich, R. J., & Rathmell, J. P. (2015). Tapering long-term opioid therapy in chronic noncancer pain: Evidence and recommendations for everyday practice. *Mayo Clinic Proceedings*, *90*(6), 828–842. https://doi.org/10.1016/j.mayocp.2015.04.003

Bohnert, A. S. B., Guy, G. P., Jr., & Losby, J. L. (2018). Opioid prescribing in the United States before and after the Centers for Disease Control and Prevention's 2016 opioid guideline. *Annals of Internal Medicine*, *169*(6), 367–375. https://doi.org/10.7326/M18-1243

Bonica, J. J. (with Loeser, J. D., Chapmann, C. R., & Fordyce, W. E.). (1990). *The management of pain* (2nd ed.). Lea & Febiger.

Brennstuhl, M.-J., Tarquinio, C., & Montel, S. (2015). Chronic pain and PTSD: Evolving views on their comorbidity. *Perspectives in Psychiatric Care*, *51*(4), 295–304. https://doi.org/10.1111/ppc.12093

Bruneau, J., Ahamad, K., Goyer, M.-È., Poulin, G., Selby, P., Fischer, B., Wild, T. C., & Wood, E. (2018). Management of opioid use disorders: A national clinical practice guideline. *CMAJ*, *190*(9), E247–E257. https://doi.org/10.1503/cmaj.170958

Buchman, D. Z., Ho, A., & Illes, J. (2016). You present like a drug addict: Patient and clinician perspectives on trust and trustworthiness in chronic pain management. *Pain Medicine*, *17*(8), 1394–1406. https://doi.org/10.1093/pm/pnv083

Bunzli, S., McEvoy, S., Dankaerts, W., O'Sullivan, P., & O'Sullivan, K. (2016). Patient perspectives on participation in cognitive functional therapy for chronic low back pain. *Physical Therapy, 96*(9), 1397–1407. https://doi.org/10.2522/ptj.20140570

Burke, A. L. J., Mathias, J. L., & Denson, L. A. (2015). Psychological functioning of people living with chronic pain: A meta-analytic review. *British Journal of Clinical Psychology, 54*(3), 345–360. https://doi.org/10.1111/bjc.12078

Butler, D. S., & Moseley, G. L. (2003). *Explain pain.* Noigroup Publications.

Butler, S. F., Budman, S. H., Fernandez, K. C., Houle, B., Benoit, C., Katz, N., & Jamison, R. N. (2007). Development and validation of the Current Opioid Misuse Measure. *Pain, 130*(1–2), 144–156. https://doi.org/10.1016/j.pain.2007.01.014

Buysse, D. J., Reynolds, C. F., III, Monk, T. H., Berman, S. R., & Kupfer, D. J. (1989). The Pittsburgh Sleep Quality Index: A new instrument for psychiatric practice and research. *Psychiatry Research, 28*(2), 193–213. https://doi.org/10.1016/0165-1781(89)90047-4

Campbell, C. M., & Edwards, R. R. (2012). Ethnic differences in pain and pain management. *Pain Management, 2*(3), 219–230. https://doi.org/10.2217/pmt.12.7

Carroll, D., & Seers, K. (1998). Relaxation for the relief of chronic pain: A systematic review. *Journal of Advanced Nursing, 27*(3), 476–487. https://doi.org/10.1046/j.1365-2648.1998.00551.x

Cavaiola, A. A., Fulmer, B. A., & Stout, D. (2015). The impact of social support and attachment style on quality of life and readiness to change in a sample of individuals receiving medication-assisted treatment for opioid dependence. *Substance Abuse, 36*(2), 183–191. https://doi.org/10.1080/08897077.2015.1019662

Center for Behavioral Health Statistics and Quality. (2018). *2017 National Survey on Drug Use and Health: Detailed tables.* Substance Abuse and Mental Health Services Administration. https://www.samhsa.gov/data/sites/default/files/cbhsq-reports/NSDUHDetailedTabs2017/NSDUHDetailedTabs2017.pdf

Centers for Disease Control and Prevention. (2015). *HAN Health advisory: Increases in fentanyl drug confiscations and fentanyl-related overdose fatalities.* http://emergency.cdc.gov/han/han00384.asp

Centers for Disease Control and Prevention. (2019). *Annual surveillance report of drug-related risks and outcomes—United States, 2019.* U.S. Department of Health and Human Services. https://www.cdc.gov/drugoverdose/pdf/pubs/2019-cdc-drug-surveillance-report.pdf

Chao, Y. S., & Ford, C. (2019). *Cognitive behavioural therapy for chronic non-cancer pain: A review of clinical effectiveness.* Canadian Agency for Drugs and Technologies in Health. https://www.ncbi.nlm.nih.gov/books/NBK549547/

Chehadi, O., Suchan, B., Konietzny, K., Köster, O., Schmidt-Wilcke, T., & Hasenbring, M. I. (2017). Gray matter alteration associated with pain catastrophizing in patients 6 months after lumbar disk surgery: A voxel-based morphometry study. *Pain Reports*, *2*(5), e617. https://doi.org/10.1097/PR9.0000000000000617

Cherkin, D. C., Sherman, K. J., Balderson, B. H., Cook, A. J., Anderson, M. L., Hawkes, R. J., Hansen, K. E., & Turner, J. A. (2016). Effect of mindfulness-based stress reduction vs cognitive behavioral therapy or usual care on back pain and functional limitations in adults with chronic low back pain: A randomized clinical trial. *JAMA*, *315*(12), 1240–1249. https://doi.org/10.1001/jama.2016.2323

Chiesa, A., & Serretti, A. (2011). Mindfulness-based interventions for chronic pain: A systematic review of the evidence. *Journal of Alternative and Complementary Medicine*, *17*(1), 83–93. https://doi.org/10.1089/acm.2009.0546

Chipidza, F. E., Wallwork, R. S., & Stern, T. A. (2015). Impact of the doctor-patient relationship. *The Primary Care Companion for CNS Disorders*, *17*(5), Article PMC4732308. https://doi.org/10.4088/PCC.15f01840

Chou, R., Deyo, R., Friedly, J., Skelly, A., Hashimoto, R., Weimer, M., Fu, R., Dana, T., Kraegel, P., Griffin, J., Grusing, S., & Brodt, E. (2016). *Noninvasive treatments for low back pain* (Comparative Effectiveness Review, No. 169). Agency for Healthcare Research and Quality. https://effectivehealthcare.ahrq.gov/sites/default/files/pdf/back-pain-treatment_research.pdf

Chou, R., Fanciullo, G. J., Fine, P. G., Adler, J. A., Ballantyne, J. C., Davies, P., Donovan, M. I., Fishbain, D. A., Foley, K. M., Fudin, J., Gilson, A. M., Kelter, A., Mauskop, A., O'Connor, P. G., Passik, S. D., Pasternak, G. W., Portenoy, R. K., Rich, B. A., Roberts, R. G., . . . Miaskowski, C. (2009). Clinical guidelines for the use of chronic opioid therapy in chronic noncancer pain. *The Journal of Pain*, *10*(2), 113–130. https://doi.org/10.1016/j.jpain.2008.10.008

Cicero, T. J., & Ellis, M. S. (2017). The prescription opioid epidemic: A review of qualitative studies on the progression from initial use to abuse. *Dialogues in Clinical Neuroscience*, *19*(3), 259–269.

Clark, M. E., Gironda, R. J., & Young, R. W. (2003). Development and validation of the Pain Outcomes Questionnaire–VA. *Journal of Rehabilitation Research and Development*, *40*(5), 381–395. https://doi.org/10.1682/JRRD.2003.09.0381

Cleeland, C. S., & Ryan, K. M. (1994). Pain assessment: Global use of the Brief Pain Inventory. *Annals of the Academy of Medicine, Singapore*, *23*(2), 129–138.

Compton, P. A., Wu, S. M., Schieffer, B., Pham, Q., & Naliboff, B. D. (2008). Introduction of a self-report version of the Prescription Drug Use Questionnaire and relationship to medication agreement noncompliance. *Journal of Pain and Symptom Management*, *36*(4), 383–395. https://doi.org/10.1016/j.jpainsymman.2007.11.006

Cook, K. F., Jensen, S. E., Schalet, B. D., Beaumont, J. L., Amtmann, D., Czajkowski, S., Dewalt, D. A., Fries, J. F., Pilkonis, P. A., Reeve, B. B., Stone, A. A., Weinfurt, K. P., & Cella, D. (2016). PROMIS measures of pain, fatigue, negative affect, physical function, and social function demonstrated clinical validity across a range of chronic conditions. *Journal of Clinical Epidemiology*, *73*, 89–102. https://doi.org/10.1016/j.jclinepi.2015.08.038

Covey, S. R. (1989). *The seven habits of highly effective people: Restoring the character ethic.* Simon & Schuster.

Cramer, H., Haller, H., Lauche, R., & Dobos, G. (2012). Mindfulness-based stress reduction for low back pain: A systematic review. *BMC Complementary and Alternative Medicine, 12,* Article 162. https://doi.org/10.1186/1472-6882-12-162

Crettaz, B., Marziniak, M., Willeke, P., Young, P., Hellhammer, D., Stumpf, A., & Burgmer, M. (2013). Stress-induced allodynia—Evidence of increased pain sensitivity in healthy humans and patients with chronic pain after experimentally induced psychosocial stress. *PLOS ONE, 8*(8), Article e69460. https://doi.org/10.1371/journal.pone.0069460

Crombez, G., Vlaeyen, J. W. S., Heuts, P. H. T. G., & Lysens, R. (1999). Fear of pain is more disabling than the pain itself: Further evidence on the role of pain-related fear in chronic back pain disability. *Pain, 80,* 329–339. https://doi.org/10.1016/S0304-3959(98)00229-2

Dahl, J., & Lundgren, T. (2006). Acceptance and commitment therapy (ACT) in the treatment of chronic pain. In R. A. Baer (Ed.), *Mindfulness-based treatment approaches: Clinician's guide to evidence base and applications* (pp. 285–306). Elsevier Academic Press.

Dakwar, E., & Levin, F. R. (2009). The emerging role of meditation in addressing psychiatric illness, with a focus on substance use disorders. *Harvard Review of Psychiatry, 17*(4), 254–267. https://doi.org/10.1080/10673220903149135

Dansie, E. J., & Turk, D. C. (2013). Assessment of patients with chronic pain. *British Journal of Anaesthesia, 111*(1), 19–25. https://doi.org/10.1093/bja/aet124

Darnall, B. D. (2018). *Psychological treatment for patients with chronic pain.* American Psychological Association.

Darnall, B. D., Mackey, S. C., Lorig, K., Kao, M.-C., Mardian, A., Stieg, R., Porter, J., DeBruyne, K., Murphy, J., Perez, L., Okvat, H., Tian, L., Flood, P., McGovern, M., Colloca, L., King, H., Van Dorsten, B., Pun, T., & Cheung, M. (2019). Comparative effectiveness of cognitive behavioral therapy for chronic pain and chronic pain self-management within the context of voluntary patient-centered prescription opioid tapering: The EMPOWER study protocol. *Pain Medicine,* pnz285. Advance online publication. https://doi.org/10.1093/pm/pnz285

Darnall, B. D., Scheman, J., Davin, S., Burns, J. W., Murphy, J. L., Wilson, A. C., Kerns, R. D., & Mackey, S. C. (2016). Pain psychology: A global needs assessment and national call to action. *Pain Medicine, 17*(2), 250–263. https://doi.org/10.1093/pm/pnv095

Darnall, B. D., Ziadni, M. S., Stieg, R. L., Mackey, I. G., Kao, M.-C., & Flood, P. (2018). Patient-centered prescription opioid tapering in community outpatients with chronic pain. *JAMA Internal Medicine, 178*(5), 707–708. https://doi.org/10.1001/jamainternmed.2017.8709

Deng, M., Chen, S.-R., Chen, H., & Pan, H.-L. (2019). α2δ-1-Bound N-Methyl-D-aspartate receptors mediate morphine-induced hyperalgesia and analgesic tolerance by potentiating glutamatergic input in rodents. *Anesthesiology*, *130*(5), 804–819. https://doi.org/10.1097/ALN.0000000000002648

Descartes, R. (1972). *Treatise of man*. Harvard University Press.

DiClemente, C. C., & Prochaska, J. O. (1982). Self-change and therapy change of smoking behavior: A comparison of processes of change in cessation and maintenance. *Addictive Behaviors*, *7*(2), 133–142. https://doi.org/10.1016/0306-4603(82)90038-7

Doran, G. T. (1981). There's a S.M.A.R.T. way to write management's goals and objectives. *Management Review*, *70*(11), 35–36.

Dowell, D., Haegerich, T. M., & Chou, R. (2016). CDC guideline for prescribing opioids for chronic pain—United States. *MMWR Recommendations and Reports*, *65*(1), 1–49. https://doi.org/10.15585/mmwr.rr6501e1

Dowell, D., Haegerich, T., & Chou, R. (2019). No shortcuts to safer opioid prescribing. *The New England Journal of Medicine*, *380*(24), 2285–2287. https://doi.org/10.1056/NEJMp1904190

Dunlay, S. M., & Strand, J. J. (2016). How to discuss goals of care with patients. *Trends in Cardiovascular Medicine*, *26*(1), 36–43. https://doi.org/10.1016/j.tcm.2015.03.018

Dworkin, R. H., Turk, D. C., Farrar, J. T., Haythornthwaite, J. A., Jensen, M. P., Katz, N. P., Kerns, R. D., Stucki, G., Allen, R. R., Bellamy, N., Carr, D. B., Chandler, J., Cowan, P., Dionne, R., Galer, B. S., Hertz, S., Jadad, A. R., Kramer, L. D., Manning, D. C., . . . Witter, J. (2005). Core outcome measures for chronic pain clinical trials: IMMPACT recommendations. *Pain*, *113*(1), 9–19. https://doi.org/10.1016/j.pain.2004.09.012

Dworkin, R. H., Turk, D. C., Wyrwich, K. W., Beaton, D., Cleeland, C. S., Farrar, J. T., Haythornthwaite, J. A., Jensen, M. P., Kerns, R. D., Ader, D. N., Brandenburg, N., Burke, L. B., Cella, D., Chandler, J., Cowan, P., Dimitrova, R., Dionne, R., Hertz, S., Jadad, A. R., . . . Zavisic, S. (2008). Interpreting the clinical importance of treatment outcomes in chronic pain clinical trials: IMMPACT recommendations. *The Journal of Pain*, *9*(2), 105–121. https://doi.org/10.1016/j.jpain.2007.09.005

Eccleston, C., & Crombez, G. (2017). Advancing psychological therapies for chronic pain. *F1000 Research*, *6*, 461. https://doi.org/10.12688/f1000research.10612.1

Eccleston, C., Fisher, E., Thomas, K. H., Hearn, L., Derry, S., Stannard, C., Knaggs, R., & Moore, R. A. (2017). Interventions for the reduction of prescribed opioid use in chronic non-cancer pain. *Cochrane Database of Systematic Reviews*. https://doi.org/10.1002/14651858.CD010323.pub3

Eccleston, C., Hearn, L., & Williams, A. C. de C. (2015). Psychological therapies for the management of chronic neuropathic pain in adults. *Cochrane Database of Systematic Reviews*. https://doi.org/10.1002/14651858.CD011259.pub2

Eccleston, C., Morley, S. J., & Williams, A. C. de C. (2013). Psychological approaches to chronic pain management: Evidence and challenges. *British Journal of Anaesthesia*, *111*(1), 59–63. https://doi.org/10.1093/bja/aet207

Edlund, M. J., Martin, B. C., Devries, A., Fan, M.-Y., Braden, J. B., & Sullivan, M. D. (2010). Trends in use of opioids for chronic noncancer pain among individuals with mental health and substance use disorders: The TROUP study. *The Clinical Journal of Pain*, *26*(1), 1–8. https://doi.org/10.1097/AJP.0b013e3181b99f35

Edwards, R. R., Dolman, A. J., Michna, E., Katz, J. N., Nedeljkovic, S. S., Janfaza, D., Isaac, Z., Martel, M. O., Jamison, R. N., & Wasan, A. D. (2016). Changes in pain sensitivity and pain modulation during oral opioid treatment: The impact of negative affect. *Pain Medicine*, *17*(10), 1882–1891. https://doi.org/10.1093/pm/pnw010

Edwards, R. R., Dworkin, R. H., Sullivan, M. D., Turk, D. C., & Wasan, A. D. (2016). The role of psychosocial processes in the development and maintenance of chronic pain. *The Journal of Pain*, *17*(Suppl. 9), T70–T92. https://doi.org/10.1016/j.jpain.2016.01.001

Ehde, D. M., Dillworth, T. M., & Turner, J. A. (2014). Cognitive-behavioral therapy for individuals with chronic pain: Efficacy, innovations, and directions for research. *American Psychologist*, *69*(2), 153–166. https://doi.org/10.1037/a0035747

Ekers, D., Richards, D., & Gilbody, S. (2008). A meta-analysis of randomized trials of behavioural treatment of depression. *Psychological Medicine*, *38*(5), 611–623. https://doi.org/10.1017/S0033291707001614

Eklund, A., De Carvalho, D., Pagé, I., Wong, A., Johansson, M. S., Pohlman, K. A., Hartvigsen, J., & Swain, M. (2019). Expectations influence treatment outcomes in patients with low back pain. A secondary analysis of data from a randomized clinical trial. *European Journal of Pain*, *23*(7), 1378–1389. https://doi.org/10.1002/ejp.1407

Ellis, A., & Velten, E. C. (1992). *When AA doesn't work for you: Rational steps to quitting alcohol*. Barricade Books Incorporated.

Engel, G. L. (1977). The need for a new medical model: A challenge for biomedicine. *Science*, *196*(4286), 129–136. https://doi.org/10.1126/science.847460

Epton, T., Currie, S., & Armitage, C. J. (2017). Unique effects of setting goals on behavior change: Systematic review and meta-analysis. *Journal of Consulting and Clinical Psychology*, *85*(12), 1182–1198. https://doi.org/10.1037/ccp0000260

Esquibel, A. Y., & Borkan, J. (2014). Doctors and patients in pain: Conflict and collaboration in opioid prescription in primary care. *Pain*, *155*(12), 2575–2582. https://doi.org/10.1016/j.pain.2014.09.018

Feingold, D., Brill, S., Goor-Aryeh, I., Delayahu, Y., & Lev-Ran, S. (2018). The association between severity of depression and prescription opioid misuse among chronic pain patients with and without anxiety: A cross-sectional study. *Journal of Affective Disorders*, *235*, 293–302. https://doi.org/10.1016/j.jad.2018.04.058

Fenton, J. J., Agnoli, A. L., Xing, G., Hang, L., Altan, A. E., Tancredi, D. J., Jerant, A., & Magnan, E. (2019). Trends and rapidity of dose tapering among patients prescribed long-term opioid therapy, 2008–2017. *JAMA Network Open, 2*(11), Article e1916271. https://doi.org/10.1001/jamanetworkopen.2019.16271

Fernandez, E., & Kerns, R. D. (2008). Anxiety, depression and anger: Core components of negative affect in medical populations. In G. J. Boyle, G. Matthews, & D. H. Saklofske (Eds.), *The Sage handbook of personality theory and testing* (Vol. 1, pp. 659–676). Sage.

Fields, H. L. (2018). How expectations influence pain. *Pain, 159*(Suppl. 1), S3–S10. https://doi.org/10.1097/j.pain.0000000000001272

Fillingim, R. B. (2017). Individual differences in pain: Understanding the mosaic that makes pain personal. *Pain, 158*(Suppl. 1), S11–S18. https://doi.org/10.1097/j.pain.0000000000000775

Fishbain, D. A., & Pulikal, A. (2019). Does opioid tapering in chronic pain patients result in improved pain or same pain vs increased pain at taper completion? A structured evidence-based systematic review. *Pain Medicine, 20*(11), 2179–2197. https://doi.org/10.1093/pm/pny231

Fisher, E., Law, E., Dudeney, J., Palermo, T. M., Stewart, G., & Eccleston, C. (2018). Psychological therapies for the management of chronic and recurrent pain in children and adolescents. *Cochrane Database of Systematic Reviews.* https://doi.org/10.1002%2F14651858.CD003968.pub5

Flor, H., Behle, D. J., & Birbaumer, N. (1993). Assessment of pain-related cognitions in chronic pain patients. *Behaviour Research and Therapy, 31*(1), 63–73. https://doi.org/10.1016/0005-7967(93)90044-U

Fordyce, W. E. (1976). *Behavioural methods for chronic pain and illness.* Mosby.

Frank, J. W., Levy, C., Matlock, D. D., Calcaterra, S. L., Mueller, S. R., Koester, S., & Binswanger, I. A. (2016). Patients' perspectives on tapering of chronic opioid therapy: A qualitative study. *Pain Medicine, 17*(10), 1838–1847. https://doi.org/10.1093/pm/pnw078

Frank, J. W., Lovejoy, T. I., Becker, W. C., Morasco, B. J., Koenig, C. J., Hoffecker, L., Dischinger, H. R., Dobscha, S. K., & Krebs, E. E. (2017). Patient outcomes in dose reduction or discontinuation of long-term opioid therapy: A systematic review. *Annals of Internal Medicine, 167*(3), 181–191. https://doi.org/10.7326/M17-0598

Gardner, P., & Oei, T. P. S. (1981). Depression and self-esteem: An investigation that used behavioral and cognitive approaches to the treatment of clinically depressed clients. *Journal of Clinical Psychology, 37*(1), 128–135. https://doi.org/10.1002/1097-4679(198101)37:1<128::AID-JCLP2270370124>3.0.CO;2-1

Garland, E. L., Brintz, C. E., Hanley, A. W., Roseen, E. J., Atchley, R. M., Gaylord, S. A., Faurot, K. R., Yaffe, J., Fiander, M., & Keefe, F. J. (2020). Mind–body therapies for opioid-treated pain: A systematic review and meta-analysis. *JAMA Internal Medicine, 180*(1), 91–105. https://doi.org/10.1001/jamainternmed.2019.4917

Gatchel, R. J. (2005). The conceptual foundations of pain management: Historical overview. In R. J. Gatchel (Ed.), *Clinical essentials of pain management* (pp. 3–18). American Psychological Association. https://doi.org/10.1037/10856-001

Gatchel, R. J., Peng, Y. B., Peters, M. L., Fuchs, P. N., & Turk, D. C. (2007). The biopsychosocial approach to chronic pain: Scientific advances and future directions. *Psychological Bulletin, 133*(4), 581–624. https://doi.org/10.1037/0033-2909.133.4.581

GBD 2015 HIV Collaborators. (2016). Estimates of global, regional, and national incidence, prevalence, and mortality of HIV, 1980–2015: The Global Burden of Disease Study 2015. *The Lancet HIV, 3*(8), e361–e387. https://doi.org/10.1016/S2352-3018(16)30087-X

Gilbert, A. L., Lee, J., Ehrlich-Jones, L., Semanik, P. A., Song, J., Pellegrini, C. A., Pinto Pt, D., Dunlop, D. D., & Chang, R. W. (2018). A randomized trial of a motivational interviewing intervention to increase lifestyle physical activity and improve self-reported function in adults with arthritis. *Seminars in Arthritis and Rheumatism, 47*(5), 732–740. https://doi.org/10.1016/j.semarthrit.2017.10.003

Gilpin, H. R., Keyes, A., Stahl, D. R., Greig, R., & McCracken, L. M. (2017). Predictors of treatment outcome in contextual cognitive and behavioral therapies for chronic pain: A systematic review. *The Journal of Pain, 18*(10), 1153–1164. https://doi.org/10.1016/j.jpain.2017.04.003

Glanz, J. M., Narwaney, K. J., Mueller, S. R., Gardner, E. M., Calcaterra, S. L., Xu, S., Breslin, K., & Binswanger, I. A. (2018). Prediction model for two-year risk of opioid overdose among patients prescribed chronic opioid therapy. *Journal of General Internal Medicine, 33*(10), 1646–1653. https://doi.org/10.1007/s11606-017-4288-3

Goesling, J., Moser, S. E., Lin, L. A., Hassett, A. L., Wasserman, R. A., & Brummett, C. M. (2018). Discrepancies between perceived benefit of opioids and self-reported patient outcomes. *Pain Medicine, 19*(2), 297–306. https://doi.org/10.1093/pm/pnw263

Gowing, L., Farrell, M., Ali, R., & White, J. M. (2016). Alpha2-adrenergic agonists for the management of opioid withdrawal. *Cochrane Database of Systematic Reviews.* https://doi.org/10.1002/14651858.CD002024.pub5

Grant, M. S., Cordts, G. A., & Doberman, D. J. (2007). Acute pain management in hospitalized patients with current opioid abuse. *Topics in Advanced Practice Nursing, 7*(1).

Greene, J., Hibbard, J. H., Alvarez, C., & Overton, V. (2016). Supporting patient behavior change: Approaches used by primary care clinicians whose patients have an increase in activation levels. *Annals of Family Medicine, 14*(2), 148–154. https://doi.org/10.1370/afm.1904

Grosscup, S. J., & Lewinsohn, P. M. (1980). Unpleasant and pleasant events, and mood. *Journal of Clinical Psychology, 36*(1), 252–259. https://doi.org/10.1002/1097-4679(198001)36:1<252::AID-JCLP2270360131>3.0.CO;2-S

Ha, J. F., & Longnecker, N. (2010). Doctor–patient communication: A review. *The Ochsner Journal, 10*(1), 38–43.

Hall, A. M., Ferreira, P. H., Maher, C. G., Latimer, J., & Ferreira, M. L. (2010). The influence of the therapist–patient relationship on treatment outcome in physical rehabilitation: A systematic review. *Physical Therapy, 90*(8), 1099–1110. https://doi.org/10.2522/ptj.20090245

Hann, K. E. J., & McCracken, L. M. (2014). A systematic review of randomized controlled trials of acceptance and commitment therapy for adults with chronic pain: Outcome domains, design quality, and efficacy. *Journal of Contextual Behavioral Science, 3*(4), 217–227. https://doi.org/10.1016/j.jcbs.2014.10.001

Harman, K., Macrae, M., Vallis, M., & Bassett, R. (2014). Working with people to make changes: A behavioural change approach used in chronic low back pain rehabilitation. *Physiotherapy Canada, 66*(1), 82–90. https://doi.org/10.3138/ptc.2012-56BC

Henry, S. G., Paterniti, D. A., Feng, B., Iosif, A.-M., Kravitz, R. L., Weinberg, G., Cowan, P., & Verba, S. (2019). Patients' experience with opioid tapering: A conceptual model with recommendations for clinicians. *The Journal of Pain, 20*(2), 181–191. https://doi.org/10.1016/j.jpain.2018.09.001

Hilton, L., Hempel, S., Ewing, B. A., Apaydin, E., Xenakis, L., Newberry, S., Colaiaco, B., Maher, A. R., Shanman, R. M., Sorbero, M. E., & Maglione, M. A. (2017). Mindfulness meditation for chronic pain: Systematic review and meta-analysis. *Annals of Behavioral Medicine, 51*(2), 199–213. https://doi.org/10.1007/s12160-016-9844-2

Howe, C. Q., & Sullivan, M. D. (2014). The missing 'P' in pain management: How the current opioid epidemic highlights the need for psychiatric services in chronic pain care. *General Hospital Psychiatry, 36*(1), 99–104. https://doi.org/10.1016/j.genhosppsych.2013.10.003

Hruschak, V., Cochran, G., & Wasan, A. D. (2018). Psychosocial interventions for chronic pain and comorbid prescription opioid use disorders: A narrative review of the literature. *Journal of Opioid Management, 14*(5), 345–358. https://doi.org/10.5055/jom.2018.0467

Hubbard, C. S., Khan, S. A., Keaser, M. L., Mathur, V. A., Goyal, M., & Seminowicz, D. A. (2014). Altered brain structure and function correlate with disease severity and pain catastrophizing in migraine patients. *eNeuro, 1*(1), ENEURO.0006-14.2014. https://doi.org/10.1523/ENEURO.0006-14.2014

Hughes, L. S., Clark, J., Colclough, J. A., Dale, E., & McMillan, D. (2017). Acceptance and commitment therapy (ACT) for chronic pain: A systematic review and meta-analyses. *The Clinical Journal of Pain, 33*(6), 552–568. https://doi.org/10.1097/AJP.0000000000000425

Hundley, L., Spradley, S., & Donelenko, S. (2018). Assessment of outcomes following high-dose opioid tapering in a Veterans Healthcare System. *Journal of Opioid Management, 14*(2), 89–101. https://doi.org/10.5055/jom.2018.0436

Ilgen, M. A., Zivin, K., McCammon, R. J., & Valenstein, M. (2008). Pain and suicidal thoughts, plans and attempts in the United States. *General Hospital Psychiatry, 30*(6), 521–527. https://doi.org/10.1016/j.genhosppsych.2008.09.003

Institute of Medicine. (2011). *Relieving pain in America: A blueprint for transforming prevention, care, education, and research.* National Academies Press.

Jackson, T., Wang, Y., Wang, Y., & Fan, H. (2014). Self-efficacy and chronic pain outcomes: A meta-analytic review. *The Journal of Pain, 15*(8), 800–814. https://doi.org/10.1016/j.jpain.2014.05.002

James, J. E., & Hardardottir, D. (2002). Influence of attention focus and trait anxiety on tolerance of acute pain. *British Journal of Health Psychology, 7*(2), 149–162. https://doi.org/10.1348/135910702169411

Jamison, R. N. (1996). *Mastering chronic pain: A professional's guide to behavioral treatment.* Professional Resource Exchange Incorporated.

Jamison, R. N., Ross, E. L., Michna, E., Chen, L. Q., Holcomb, C., & Wasan, A. D. (2010). Substance misuse treatment for high-risk chronic pain patients on opioid therapy: A randomized trial. *Pain, 150*(3), 390–400. https://doi.org/10.1016/j.pain.2010.02.033

Jensen, M. P., Gianas, A., Sherlin, L. H., & Howe, J. D. (2015). Pain catastrophizing and EEG-alpha asymmetry. *The Clinical Journal of Pain, 31*(10), 852–858. https://doi.org/10.1097/AJP.0000000000000182

Jensen, M. P., & Karoly, P. (2001). Self-report scales and procedures for assessing pain in adults. In D. C. Turk & R. Melzack (Eds.), *Handbook of pain assessment* (pp. 15–34). Guilford Press.

Jensen, M. P., Karoly, P., & Braver, S. (1986). The measurement of clinical pain intensity: A comparison of six methods. *Pain, 27*(1), 117–126. https://doi.org/10.1016/0304-3959(86)90228-9

Jensen, M. P., Turner, J. A., Romano, J. M., & Strom, S. E. (1995). The Chronic Pain Coping Inventory: Development and preliminary validation. *Pain, 60*(2), 203–216. https://doi.org/10.1016/0304-3959(94)00118-X

Johnson, K., Jones, C., Compton, W., Baldwin, G., Fan, J., Mermin, J., & Bennett, J. (2018). Federal response to the opioid crisis. *Current HIV/AIDS Reports, 15*(4), 293–301. https://doi.org/10.1007/s11904-018-0398-8

Johnson, M. H., Breakwell, G., Douglas, W., & Humphries, S. (1998). The effects of imagery and sensory detection distractors on different measures of pain: How does distraction work? *British Journal of Clinical Psychology, 37*(2), 141–154. https://doi.org/10.1111/j.2044-8260.1998.tb01290.x

Juurlink, D. N. (2017). Rethinking "doing well" on chronic opioid therapy. *CMAJ, 189*(39), E1222–E1223. https://doi.org/10.1503/cmaj.170628

Kabat-Zinn, J. (1982). An outpatient program in behavioral medicine for chronic pain patients based on the practice of mindfulness meditation: Theoretical considerations and preliminary results. *General Hospital Psychiatry, 4*(1), 33–47. https://doi.org/10.1016/0163-8343(82)90026-3

Kabat-Zinn, J. (1990). *Full catastrophe living: Using the wisdom of your body and mind to face stress, pain and illness.* Delacorte.

Kabat-Zinn, J. (2003). Mindfulness-based interventions in context: Past, present, and future. *Clinical Psychology: Science and Practice, 10*(2), 144–156. https://doi.org/10.1093/clipsy.bpg016

Kampman, K., & Jarvis, M. (2015). American Society of Addiction Medicine (ASAM) national practice guideline for the use of medications in the treatment of addiction involving opioid use. *Journal of Addiction Medicine, 9*(5), 358–367. https://doi.org/10.1097/ADM.0000000000000166

Kanji, N. (2000). Management of pain through autogenic training. *Complementary Therapies in Nursing & Midwifery, 6*(3), 143–148. https://doi.org/10.1054/ctnm.2000.0473

Keefe, F. J., & Van Horn, Y. (1993). Cognitive-behavioral treatment of rheumatoid arthritis pain: Maintaining treatment gains. *Arthritis Care and Research, 6*(4), 213–222. https://doi.org/10.1002/art.1790060408

Kelley, J. M., Kraft-Todd, G., Schapira, L., Kossowsky, J., & Riess, H. (2014). The influence of the patient–clinician relationship on healthcare outcomes: A systematic review and meta-analysis of randomized controlled trials. *PLOS ONE, 9*(4), Article e94207. https://doi.org/10.1371/journal.pone.0094207

Kellezi, B., Coupland, C., Morriss, R., Beckett, K., Joseph, S., Barnes, J., Christie, N., Sleney, J., & Kendrick, D. (2017). The impact of psychological factors on recovery from injury: A multicentre cohort study. *Social Psychiatry and Psychiatric Epidemiology, 52*(7), 855–866. https://doi.org/10.1007/s00127-016-1299-z

Kelly, J. F., Dow, S. J., & Westerhoff, C. (2010). Does our choice of substance-related terms influence perceptions of treatment need? An empirical investigation with two commonly used terms. *Journal of Drug Issues, 40*(4), 805–818. https://doi.org/10.1177/002204261004000403

Kelly, M. P., & Barker, M. (2016). Why is changing health-related behaviour so difficult? *Public Health, 136*, 109–116. https://doi.org/10.1016/j.puhe.2016.03.030

Kerns, R. D., Rosenberg, R., Jamison, R. N., Caudill, M. A., & Haythornthwaite, J. (1997). Readiness to adopt a self-management approach to chronic pain: The Pain Stages of Change Questionnaire (PSOCQ). *Pain, 72*(1–2), 227–234. https://doi.org/10.1016/S0304-3959(97)00038-9

Kerns, R. D., Turk, D. C., & Rudy, T. E. (1985). The West Haven–Yale Multidimensional Pain Inventory (WHYMPI). *Pain*, *23*(4), 345–356. https://doi.org/10.1016/0304-3959(85)90004-1

Kinney, M., Seider, J., Beaty, A. F., Coughlin, K., Dyal, M., & Clewley, D. (2018). The impact of therapeutic alliance in physical therapy for chronic musculoskeletal pain: A systematic review of the literature. *Physiotherapy Theory and Practice*, 1–13. https://doi.org/10.1080/09593985.2018.1516015

Knoerl, R., Lavoie Smith, E. M., & Weisberg, J. (2016). Chronic pain and cognitive behavioral therapy: An integrative review. *Western Journal of Nursing Research*, *38*(5), 596–628. https://doi.org/10.1177/0193945915615869

Krebs, E. E., Gravely, A., Nugent, S., Jensen, A. C., DeRonne, B., Goldsmith, E. S., Kroenke, K., Bair, M. J., & Noorbaloochi, S. (2018). Effect of opioid vs nonopioid medications on pain-related function in patients with chronic back pain or hip or knee osteoarthritis pain: The SPACE randomized clinical trial. *JAMA*, *319*(9), 872–882. https://doi.org/10.1001/jama.2018.0899

Krebs, E. E., Lorenz, K. A., Bair, M. J., Damush, T. M., Wu, J., Sutherland, J. M., Asch, S. M., & Kroenke, K. (2009). Development and initial validation of the PEG, a three-item scale assessing pain intensity and interference. *Journal of General Internal Medicine*, *24*(6), 733–738. https://doi.org/10.1007/s11606-009-0981-1

Kresina, T. F., & Lubran, R. (2011). Improving public health through access to and utilization of medication assisted treatment. *International Journal of Environmental Research and Public Health*, *8*(10), 4102–4117. https://doi.org/10.3390/ijerph8104102

Kroenke, K. (2018). Pain measurement in research and practice. *Journal of General Internal Medicine*, *33*(Suppl. 1), 7–8. https://doi.org/10.1007/s11606-018-4363-4

Kroenke, K., Spitzer, R. L., & Williams, J. B. W. (2002). The PHQ-15: Validity of a new measure for evaluating the severity of somatic symptoms. *Psychosomatic Medicine*, *64*(2), 258–266. https://doi.org/10.1097/00006842-200203000-00008

Kübler-Ross, E. (1973). *On death and dying*. Routledge. https://doi.org/10.4324/9780203010495

Kwasnicka, D., Dombrowski, S. U., White, M., & Sniehotta, F. (2016). Theoretical explanations for maintenance of behaviour change: A systematic review of behaviour theories. *Health Psychology Review*, *10*(3), 277–296. https://doi.org/10.1080/17437199.2016.1151372

Kwekkeboom, K. L., Cherwin, C. H., Lee, J. W., & Wanta, B. (2010). Mind-body treatments for the pain–fatigue–sleep disturbance symptom cluster in persons with cancer. *Journal of Pain and Symptom Management*, *39*(1), 126–138. https://doi.org/10.1016/j.jpainsymman.2009.05.022

Lauche, R., Cramer, H., Dobos, G., Langhorst, J., & Schmidt, S. (2013). A systematic review and meta-analysis of mindfulness-based stress reduction for the fibromyalgia syndrome. *Journal of Psychosomatic Research*, *75*(6), 500–510. https://doi.org/10.1016/j.jpsychores.2013.10.010

Lawrence, J. M., Hoeft, F., Sheau, K. E., & Mackey, S. C. (2011). Strategy-dependent dissociation of the neural correlates involved in pain modulation. *Anesthesiology*, *115*(4), 844–851. https://doi.org/10.1097/ALN. 0b013e31822b79ea

Lee, M., Silverman, S. M., Hansen, H., Patel, V. B., & Manchikanti, L. (2011). A comprehensive review of opioid-induced hyperalgesia. *Pain Physician*, *14*(2), 145–161.

Lerman, S. F., Rudich, Z., Brill, S., Shalev, H., & Shahar, G. (2015). Longitudinal associations between depression, anxiety, pain, and pain-related disability in chronic pain patients. *Psychosomatic Medicine*, *77*(3), 333–341. https:// doi.org/10.1097/PSY.0000000000000158

Lewinsohn, P. M., Muñoz, R. F., Youngren, M. A., & Zeiss, A. M. (1978). *Control your depression*. Prentice-Hall.

Linde, K., Witt, C. M., Streng, A., Weidenhammer, W., Wagenpfeil, S., Brinkhaus, B., Willich, S. N., & Melchart, D. (2007). The impact of patient expectations on outcomes in four randomized controlled trials of acupuncture in patients with chronic pain. *Pain*, *128*(3), 264–271. https://doi.org/ 10.1016/j.pain.2006.12.006

Linton, S. J., & Bergbom, S. (2011). Understanding the link between depression and pain. *Scandinavian Journal of Pain*, *2*(2), 47–54. https://doi.org/10.1016/ j.sjpain.2011.01.005

Logsdon, R. G., McCurry, S. M., & Teri, L. (2007). Evidence-based interventions to improve quality of life for individuals with dementia. *Alzheimer's Care Today*, *8*(4), 309–318. https://www.ncbi.nlm.nih.gov/pmc/articles/PMC2585781/

Malouff, J. M., Thorsteinsson, E. B., & Schutte, N. S. (2007). The efficacy of problem solving therapy in reducing mental and physical health problems: A meta-analysis. *Clinical Psychology Review*, *27*(1), 46–57. https://doi.org/ 10.1016/j.cpr.2005.12.005

Manchikanti, L., Giordano, J., Boswell, M. V., Fellows, B., Manchukonda, R., & Pampati, V. (2007). Psychological factors as predictors of opioid abuse and illicit drug use in chronic pain patients. *Journal of Opioid Management*, *3*(2), 89–100. https://doi.org/10.5055/jom.2007.0045

Manhapra, A., Arias, A. J., & Ballantyne, J. C. (2018). The conundrum of opioid tapering in long-term opioid therapy for chronic pain: A commentary. *Substance Abuse*, *39*(2), 152–161. https://doi.org/10.1080/08897077.2017.1381663

Mankovsky, T., Lynch, M., Clark, A., Sawynok, J., & Sullivan, M. J. (2012). Pain catastrophizing predicts poor response to topical analgesics in patients with neuropathic pain. *Pain Research & Management*, *17*(1), 10–14. https:// doi.org/10.1155/2012/970423

Markland, D., Ryan, R. M., Tobin, V. J., & Rollnick, S. (2005). Motivational interviewing and self-determination theory. *Journal of Social and Clinical Psychology*, *24*(6), 811–831. https://doi.org/10.1521/jscp.2005.24.6.811

Maroon, J. C., Bost, J. W., & Maroon, A. (2010). Natural anti-inflammatory agents for pain relief. *Surgical Neurology International, 1*, 80.

Martel, M. O., Wasan, A. D., Jamison, R. N., & Edwards, R. R. (2013). Catastrophic thinking and increased risk for prescription opioid misuse in patients with chronic pain. *Drug and Alcohol Dependence, 132*(1–2), 335–341. https://doi.org/10.1016/j.drugalcdep.2013.02.034

Martino, J. G., Smith, S. R., Rafie, S., Rafie, S., & Marienfeld, C. (2020). Physician and pharmacist: Attitudes, facilitators, and barriers to prescribing naloxone for home rescue. *The American Journal on Addictions, 29*(1), 65–72. https://doi.org/10.1111/ajad.12982

Matthewson, G., Woo, C.-W., Reddan, M. C., & Wager, T. D. (2019). Cognitive self-regulation influences pain-related physiology. *Pain, 160*(10), 2338–2349. https://doi.org/10.1097/j.pain.0000000000001621

Mazzucchelli, T. G., Kane, R. T., & Rees, C. S. (2010). Behavioral activation interventions for well-being: A meta-analysis. *The Journal of Positive Psychology, 5*(2), 105–121. https://doi.org/10.1080/17439760903569154

McCracken, L. M., & Vowles, K. E. (2014). Acceptance and commitment therapy and mindfulness for chronic pain: Model, process, and progress. *American Psychologist, 69*(2), 178–187. https://doi.org/10.1037/a0035623

McHugh, R. K., Weiss, R. D., Cornelius, M., Martel, M. O., Jamison, R. N., & Edwards, R. R. (2016). Distress intolerance and prescription opioid misuse among patients with chronic pain. *The Journal of Pain, 17*(7), 806–814. https://doi.org/10.1016/j.jpain.2016.03.004

McNair, D. M., Lorr, M., & Droppelman, L. F. (1971). *POMS: Manual for the profile of mood states*. Educational and Industrial Testing Service.

Melzack, R. (1999). Pain and stress: A new perspective. In R. J. Gatchel & D. C. Turk (Eds.), *Psychosocial factors in pain: Critical perspectives* (pp. 89–106). Guilford Press.

Melzack, R. (2001). Pain and the neuromatrix in the brain. *Journal of Dental Education, 65*(12), 1378–1382.

Melzack, R., & Wall, P. D. (1965). Pain mechanisms: A new theory. *Science, 150*(3699), 971–979. https://doi.org/10.1126/science.150.3699.971

Miller, W. R. (1995). *Motivational enhancement therapy manual: A clinical research guide for therapists treating individuals with alcohol abuse and dependence*. Diane Publishing.

Miller, W. R., & Rollnick, S. (1991). *Motivational interviewing. Preparing people to change addictive behavior*. Guilford Press.

Miller, W. R., & Rollnick, S. (2002). *Motivational interviewing: Preparing people for change* (2nd ed.). Guilford Press.

Moayedi, M., & Davis, K. D. (2013). Theories of pain: From specificity to gate control. *Journal of Neurophysiology, 109*(1), 5–12. https://doi.org/10.1152/jn.00457.2012

Mojtabai, R. (2018). National trends in long-term use of prescription opioids. *Pharmacoepidemiology and Drug Safety, 27*(5), 526–534. https://doi.org/10.1002/pds.4278

Moldofsky, H. (2001). Sleep and pain. *Sleep Medicine Reviews, 5*(5), 385–396. https://doi.org/10.1053/smrv.2001.0179

Morasco, B. J., O'Hearn, D., Turk, D. C., & Dobscha, S. K. (2014). Associations between prescription opioid use and sleep impairment among veterans with chronic pain. *Pain Medicine, 15*(11), 1902–1910. https://doi.org/10.1111/pme.12472

Morgan, M. M., & Christie, M. J. (2011). Analysis of opioid efficacy, tolerance, addiction and dependence from cell culture to human. *British Journal of Pharmacology, 164*(4), 1322–1334. https://doi.org/10.1111/j.1476-5381.2011.01335.x

Morin, C. M., Belleville, G., Bélanger, L., & Ivers, H. (2011). The Insomnia Severity Index: Psychometric indicators to detect insomnia cases and evaluate treatment response. *Sleep, 34*(5), 601–608. https://doi.org/10.1093/sleep/34.5.601

Morley, S., Eccleston, C., & Williams, A. (1999). Systematic review and meta-analysis of randomized controlled trials of cognitive behaviour therapy and behaviour therapy for chronic pain in adults, excluding headache. *Pain, 80*(1–2), 1–13. https://doi.org/10.1016/S0304-3959(98)00255-3

Morone, N. E., Greco, C. M., Moore, C. G., Rollman, B. L., Lane, B., Morrow, L. A., Glynn, N. W., & Weiner, D. K. (2016). A mind-body program for older adults with chronic low back pain: A randomized clinical trial. *JAMA Internal Medicine, 176*(3), 329–337. https://doi.org/10.1001/jamainternmed.2015.8033

Murphy, J. L., Clark, M. E., & Banou, E. (2013). Opioid cessation and multidimensional outcomes after interdisciplinary chronic pain treatment. *The Clinical Journal of Pain, 29*(2), 109–117. https://doi.org/10.1097/AJP.0b013e3182579935

Murphy, J. L., McKellar, J. M., Raffa, S. D., Clark, M. E., Kerns, R. D., & Karlin, B. E. (2014). *Cognitive behavioral therapy for chronic pain among veterans: Therapist manual*. Department of Veterans Affairs. https://www.va.gov/PAINMANAGEMENT/docs/CBT-CP_Therapist_Manual.pdf

Murphy, J. L., Phillips, K. M., & Rafie, S. (2016). Sex differences between Veterans participating in interdisciplinary chronic pain rehabilitation. *Journal of Rehabilitation Research and Development, 53*(1), 83–94. https://doi.org/10.1682/JRRD.2014.10.0250

National Academies of Sciences, Engineering, and Medicine. (2017). *Pain management and the opioid epidemic: Balancing societal and individual benefits and risks of prescription opioid use*. The National Academies Press. https://doi.org/10.17226/24781

National Academies of Sciences, Engineering, and Medicine. (2018). *Medication-assisted treatment for opioid use disorder: Proceedings of a workshop—in brief.* The National Academies Press. https://doi.org/10.17226/25322

National Center for Health Statistics. (2020). *Multiple cause of death, 1999–2018* [Data set]. CDC WONDER Online Database. http://wonder.cdc.gov/mcd-icd10.html

National Center for Injury Prevention and Control. (n.d.). *Opioid basics: Commonly used terms.* https://www.cdc.gov/drugoverdose/opioids/terms.html

Naylor, M. R., Naud, S., Keefe, F. J., & Helzer, J. E. (2010). Therapeutic interactive voice response (TIVR) to reduce analgesic medication use for chronic pain management. *The Journal of Pain, 11*(12), 1410–1419. https://doi.org/10.1016/j.jpain.2010.03.019

Nicassio, P. M., & Wallston, K. A. (1992). Longitudinal relationships among pain, sleep problems, and depression in rheumatoid arthritis. *Journal of Abnormal Psychology, 101*(3), 514–520. https://doi.org/10.1037/0021-843X.101.3.514

Nicholas, M. K. (1989). *Self-efficacy and chronic pain* [Paper presentation]. Annual Conference of the British Psychological Society, St. Andrews.

Nicholas, M. K. (2007). The pain self-efficacy questionnaire: Taking pain into account. *European Journal of Pain, 11*(2), 153–163. https://doi.org/10.1016/j.ejpain.2005.12.008

Nielson, W. R., Armstrong, J. M., Jensen, M. P., & Kerns, R. D. (2009). Two brief versions of the Multidimensional Pain Readiness to Change Questionnaire, Version 2 (MPRCQ2). *The Clinical Journal of Pain, 25*(1), 48–57. https://doi.org/10.1097/AJP.0b013e3181817ab4

Nielson, W. R., Jensen, M. P., Ehde, D. M., Kerns, R. D., & Molton, I. R. (2008). Further development of the Multidimensional Pain Readiness to Change Questionnaire: The MPRCQ2. *The Journal of Pain, 9*(6), 552–565. https://doi.org/10.1016/j.jpain.2008.01.327

Nielson, W. R., Jensen, M. P., & Kerns, R. D. (2003). Initial development and validation of a Multidimensional Pain Readiness to Change Questionnaire. *The Journal of Pain, 4*(3), 148–158. https://doi.org/10.1054/jpai.2003.436

Oliva, E. M., Bowe, T., Manhapra, A., Kertesz. S., Hah, J. M., Henderson, P., Robinson, A., Paik, M., Sandbrink, F., Gordon, A. J., & Trafton, J. A. (2020). Associations between stopping prescriptions for opioids, length of treatment, and overdose or suicide deaths in U.S. veterans: Observational evaluation. *BMJ, 368*(8236), m283. https://doi.org/10.1136/bmj.m283

Ory, M. G., Lee Smith, M., Mier, N., & Wernicke, M. M. (2010). The science of sustaining health behavior change: The health maintenance consortium. *American Journal of Health Behavior, 34*(6), 647–659. https://doi.org/10.5993/AJHB.34.6.2

Palermo, T. M. (2012). *Cognitive-behavioral therapy for chronic pain in children and adolescents.* Oxford University Press.

Panchal, S. J., Müller-Schwefe, P., & Wurzelmann, J. I. (2007). Opioid-induced bowel dysfunction: Prevalence, pathophysiology and burden. *International Journal of Clinical Practice, 61*(7), 1181–1187. https://doi.org/10.1111/j.1742-1241.2007.01415.x

Penney, L. S., Ritenbaugh, C., DeBar, L. L., Elder, C., & Deyo, R. A. (2017). Provider and patient perspectives on opioids and alternative treatments for managing chronic pain: A qualitative study. *BMC Family Practice, 17*, Article 164. https://doi.org/10.1186/s12875-016-0566-0

Petrosky, E., Harpaz, R., Fowler, K. A., Bohm, M. K., Helmick, C. G., Yuan, K., & Betz, C. J. (2018). Chronic pain among suicide decedents, 2003 to 2014: Findings from the National Violent Death Reporting System. *Annals of Internal Medicine, 169*(7), 448–455. https://doi.org/10.7326/M18-0830

Ploghaus, A., Narain, C., Beckmann, C. F., Clare, S., Bantick, S., Wise, R., Matthews, P. M., Rawlins, J. N., & Tracey, I. (2001). Exacerbation of pain by anxiety is associated with activity in a hippocampal network. *The Journal of Neuroscience, 21*(24), 9896–9903. https://doi.org/10.1523/JNEUROSCI.21.24.09896.2001

Prochaska, J. O., & DiClemente, C. C. (1982). Transtheoretical therapy: Toward a more integrative model of change. *Psychotherapy: Theory, Research, & Practice, 19*(3), 276–288. https://doi.org/10.1037/h0088437

Quartana, P. J., Campbell, C. M., & Edwards, R. R. (2009). Pain catastrophizing: A critical review. *Expert Review of Neurotherapeutics, 9*(5), 745–758. https://doi.org/10.1586/ern.09.34

Raymond, I., Ancoli-Israel, S., & Choinière, M. (2004). Sleep disturbances, pain and analgesia in adults hospitalized for burn injuries. *Sleep Medicine, 5*(6), 551–559. https://doi.org/10.1016/j.sleep.2004.07.007

Reiner, K., Tibi, L., & Lipsitz, J. D. (2013). Do mindfulness-based interventions reduce pain intensity? A critical review of the literature. *Pain Medicine, 14*(2), 230–242. https://doi.org/10.1111/pme.12006

Revicki, D. A., Chen, W.-H., Harnam, N., Cook, K. F., Amtmann, D., Callahan, L. F., Jensen, M. P., & Keefe, F. J. (2009). Development and psychometric analysis of the PROMIS pain behavior item bank. *Pain, 146*(1–2), 158–169. https://doi.org/10.1016/j.pain.2009.07.029

Rey, R. (1989). *The history of pain*. Harvard University Press.

Richmond, H., Hall, A. M., Copsey, B., Hansen, Z., Williamson, E., Hoxey-Thomas, N., Cooper, Z., & Lamb, S. E. (2015). The effectiveness of cognitive behavioural treatment for non-specific low back pain: A systematic review and meta-analysis. *PLOS ONE, 10*(8), e0134192. https://doi.org/10.1371/journal.pone.0134192

Roditi, D., & Robinson, M. E. (2011). The role of psychological interventions in the management of patients with chronic pain. *Psychology Research and Behavior Management, 4*, 41–49. https://doi.org/10.2147/PRBM.S15375

Rogers, C. R. (1946). Significant aspects of client-centered therapy. *American Psychologist, 1*(10), 415–422. https://doi.org/10.1037/h0060866

Rose, M. J., Reilly, J. P., Pennie, B., Bowen-Jones, K., Stanley, I. M., & Slade, P. D. (1997). Chronic low back pain rehabilitation programs: A study of the optimum duration of treatment and a comparison of group and individual therapy. *Spine, 22*(19), 2246–2251. https://doi.org/10.1097/00007632-199710010-00009

Rosen, I. M., Aurora, R. N., Kirsch, D. B., Carden, K. A., Malhotra, R. K., Ramar, K., Abbasi-Feinberg, F., Kristo, D. A., Martin, J. L., Olson, E. J., Rosen, C. L., Rowley, J. A., Shelgikar, A. V., & the American Academy of Sleep Medicine Board of Directors. (2019). Chronic opioid therapy and sleep: An American Academy of Sleep Medicine position statement. *Journal of Clinical Sleep Medicine, 15*(11), 1671–1673. https://doi.org/10.5664/jcsm.8062

Rummans, T. A., Burton, M. C., & Dawson, N. L. (2018). How good intentions contributed to bad outcomes: The opioid crisis. *Mayo Clinic Proceedings, 93*(3), 344–350. https://doi.org/10.1016/j.mayocp.2017.12.020

Rupp, T., & Delaney, K. A. (2004). Inadequate analgesia in emergency medicine. *Annals of Emergency Medicine, 43*(4), 494–503. https://doi.org/10.1016/j.annemergmed.2003.11.019

Salamon, E., Esch, T., & Stefano, G. B. (2006). Pain and relaxation (review). *International Journal of Molecular Medicine, 18*(3), 465–470.

Sandhu, H. K., Abraham, C., Alleyne, S., Balasubramanian, S., Betteley, L., Booth, K., Carnes, D., Furlan, A. D., Haywood, K., Iglesias Urrutia, C. P., Lall, R., Manca, A., Mistry, D., Nichols, V. P., Noyes, J., Rahman, A., Seers, K., Shaw, J., Tang, N. K. Y., . . . Eldabe, S. (2019). Testing a support programme for opioid reduction for people with chronic non-malignant pain: The I-WOTCH randomised controlled trial protocol. *BMJ Open, 9*(8), e028937.

Santoro, T. N., & Santoro, J. D. (2018). Racial BIAS in the US opioid epidemic: A review of the history of systemic bias and implications for care. *Cureus, 10*(12), e3733. https://doi.org/10.7759/cureus.3733

Scherrer, J. F., Salas, J., Copeland, L. A., Stock, E. M., Ahmedani, B. K., Sullivan, M. D., Burroughs, T., Schneider, F. D., Bucholz, K. K., & Lustman, P. J. (2016). Prescription opioid duration, dose, and increased risk of depression in 3 large patient populations. *Annals of Family Medicine, 14*(1), 54–62. https://doi.org/10.1370/afm.1885

Schütze, R., Rees, C., Smith, A., Slater, H., Campbell, J. M., & O'Sullivan, P. (2018). How can we best reduce pain catastrophizing in adults with chronic noncancer pain? A systematic review and meta-analysis. *The Journal of Pain, 19*(3), 233–256. https://doi.org/10.1016/j.jpain.2017.09.010

Seaman, D. R. (2012). Anti-inflammatory diet for pain patients. *Practical Pain Management, 12*(10), 36–46. https://www.practicalpainmanagement.com/treatments/complementary/anti-inflammatory-diet-pain-patients?page=0,2

Seminowicz, D. A., & Davis, K. D. (2006). Cortical responses to pain in healthy individuals depends on pain catastrophizing. *Pain, 120*(3), 297–306. https://doi.org/10.1016/j.pain.2005.11.008

Seminowicz, D. A., Shpaner, M., Keaser, M. L., Krauthamer, G. M., Mantegna, J., Dumas, J. A., Newhouse, P. A., Filippi, C. G., Keefe, F. J., & Naylor, M. R. (2013). Cognitive-behavioral therapy increases prefrontal cortex gray matter in patients with chronic pain. *The Journal of Pain, 14*(12), 1573–1584. https://doi.org/10.1016/j.jpain.2013.07.020

Sherman, K. J., Walker, R. L., Saunders, K., Shortreed, S. M., Parchman, M., Hansen, R. N., Thakral, M., Ludman, E. J., Dublin, S., & Von Korff, M. (2018). Doctor–patient trust among chronic pain patients on chronic opioid therapy after opioid risk reduction initiatives: A survey. *Journal of the American Board of Family Medicine, 31*(4), 578–587. https://doi.org/10.3122/jabfm.2018.04.180021

Shpaner, M., Kelly, C., Lieberman, G., Perelman, H., Davis, M., Keefe, F. J., & Naylor, M. R. (2014). Unlearning chronic pain: A randomized controlled trial to investigate changes in intrinsic brain connectivity following cognitive behavioral therapy. *NeuroImage: Clinical, 5*, 365–376. https://doi.org/10.1016/j.nicl.2014.07.008

Skelly, A. C., Chou, R., Dettori, J. R., Turner, J. A., Friedly, J. L., Rundell, S. D., Fu, R., Brodt, E. D., Wasson, N., Winter, C., & Ferguson, A. J. R. (2018). *Noninvasive nonpharmacological treatment for chronic pain: A systematic review.* Agency for Healthcare Research and Quality. https://doi.org/10.23970/AHRQEPCCER209

Skinner, B. F. (1965). *Science and human behavior.* Free Press.

Speed, T. J., Parekh, V., Coe, W., & Antoine, D. (2018). Comorbid chronic pain and opioid use disorder: Literature review and potential treatment innovations. *International Review of Psychiatry, 30*(5), 136–146. https://doi.org/10.1080/09540261.2018.1514369

Spitzer, R. L., Kroenke, K., Williams, J. B. W., & Löwe, B. (2006). A brief measure for assessing generalized anxiety disorder: The GAD-7. *Archives of Internal Medicine, 166*(10), 1092–1097. https://doi.org/10.1001/archinte.166.10.1092

Stevens, M. J., & Lane, A. M. (2001). Mood-regulating strategies used by athletes. *Athletic Insight, 3*(3), 1–12. https://pdfs.semanticscholar.org/947b/d19cbc7761b88316fbf9c3e04e712f6d3382.pdf

Stewart, M. O., Karlin, B. E., Murphy, J. L., Raffa, S. D., Miller, S. A., McKellar, J., & Kerns, R. D. (2015). National dissemination of cognitive-behavioral therapy for chronic pain in veterans: Therapist and patient-level outcomes. *The Clinical Journal of Pain, 31*(8), 722–729. https://doi.org/10.1097/AJP.0000000000000151

Strunin, L., & Boden, L. I. (2004). Family consequences of chronic back pain. *Social Science & Medicine, 58*(7), 1385–1393. https://doi.org/10.1016/S0277-9536(03)00333-2

Sturgeon, J. A. (2014). Psychological therapies for the management of chronic pain. *Psychology Research and Behavior Management, 7*, 115–124. https://doi.org/10.2147/PRBM.S44762

Sullivan, M. D. (2010). Who gets high-dose opioid therapy for chronic non-cancer pain? *Pain, 151*(3), 567–568. https://doi.org/10.1016/j.pain.2010.08.036

Sullivan, M. D., & Howe, C. Q. (2013). Opioid therapy for chronic pain in the United States: Promises and perils. *Pain, 154*(Suppl. 1), S94–S100. https://doi.org/10.1016/j.pain.2013.09.009

Sullivan, M. D., Turner, J. A., DiLodovico, C., D'Appollonio, A., Stephens, K., & Chan, Y.-F. (2017). Prescription opioid taper support for outpatients with chronic pain: A randomized controlled trial. *The Journal of Pain, 18*(3), 308–318. https://doi.org/10.1016/j.jpain.2016.11.003

Sullivan, M. J., Thorn, B., Haythornthwaite, J. A., Keefe, F., Martin, M., Bradley, L. A., & Lefebvre, J. C. (2001). Theoretical perspectives on the relation between catastrophizing and pain. *The Clinical Journal of Pain, 17*(1), 52–64. https://doi.org/10.1097/00002508-200103000-00008

Sullivan, M. J. L., Bishop, S. R., & Pivik, J. (1995). The Pain Catastrophizing Scale: Development and validation. *Psychological Assessment, 7*(4), 524–532. https://doi.org/10.1037/1040-3590.7.4.524

Swegle, J. M., & Logemann, C. (2006). Management of common opioid-induced adverse effects. *American Family Physician, 74*(8), 1347–1354.

Tang, N. K. Y., & Crane, C. (2006). Suicidality in chronic pain: A review of the prevalence, risk factors and psychological links. *Psychological Medicine, 36*(5), 575–586. https://doi.org/10.1017/S0033291705006859

Thibault, P., Loisel, P., Durand, M.-J., Catchlove, R., & Sullivan, M. J. L. (2008). Psychological predictors of pain expression and activity intolerance in chronic pain patients. *Pain, 139*(1), 47–54. https://doi.org/10.1016/j.pain.2008.02.029

Thomas, M. L., Elliott, J. E., Rao, S. M., Fahey, K. F., Paul, S. M., & Miaskowski, C. (2012). A randomized, clinical trial of education or motivational-interviewing-based coaching compared to usual care to improve cancer pain management. *Oncology Nursing Forum, 39*(1), 39–49. https://doi.org/10.1188/12.ONF.39-49

Tota-Faucette, M. E., Gil, K. M., Williams, D. A., Keefe, F. J., & Goli, V. (1993). Predictors of response to pain management treatment. The role of family environment and changes in cognitive processes. *The Clinical Journal of Pain, 9*, 115–123. https://doi.org/10.1097/00002508-199306000-00006

Toth, C., Brady, S., & Hatfield, M. (2014). The importance of catastrophizing for successful pharmacological treatment of peripheral neuropathic pain. *Journal of Pain Research, 7*, 327–338. https://doi.org/10.2147/JPR.S56883

Toye, F., Seers, K., Tierney, S., & Barker, K. L. (2017). A qualitative evidence synthesis to explore healthcare professionals' experience of prescribing opioids to adults with chronic non-malignant pain. *BMC Family Practice, 18*, Article 94. https://doi.org/10.1186/s12875-017-0663-8

Tse, M. M. Y., Vong, S. K. S., & Tang, S. K. (2013). Motivational interviewing and exercise programme for community-dwelling older persons with chronic pain: A randomised controlled study. *Journal of Clinical Nursing, 22*(13–14), 1843–1856. https://doi.org/10.1111/j.1365-2702.2012.04317.x

Turk, D. C., & Monarch, E. S. (2002). Biopsychosocial perspective on chronic pain. In D. C. Turk & R. J. Gatchel (Eds.), *Psychological approaches to pain management: A practitioner's handbook* (pp. 3–29). Guilford Press.

Turk, D. C., & Robinson, J. P. (2011). Assessment of patients with chronic pain: A comprehensive approach. In D. C. Turk & R. Melzack (Eds.), *Handbook of pain assessment* (3rd ed., pp. 188–210). Guilford Press.

Turk, D. C., Swanson, K. S., & Gatchel, R. J. (2008). Predicting opioid misuse by chronic pain patients: A systematic review and literature synthesis. *The Clinical Journal of Pain, 24*(6), 497–508. https://doi.org/10.1097/AJP.0b013e31816b1070

Upshur, C. C., Bacigalupe, G., & Luckmann, R. (2010). "They don't want anything to do with you": Patient views of primary care management of chronic pain. *Pain Medicine, 11*(12), 1791–1798. https://doi.org/10.1111/j.1526-4637.2010.00960.x

U.S. Department of Health and Human Services. (2019a). *HHS guide for clinicians on the appropriate dosage reduction or discontinuation of long-term opioid analgesics.* https://www.hhs.gov/opioids/sites/default/files/2019 10/Dosage_Reduction_Discontinuation.pdf

U.S. Department of Health and Human Services. (2019b). *Pain management best practices inter-agency task force report: Updates, gaps, inconsistencies, and recommendations.* https://www.hhs.gov/ash/advisory-committees/pain/reports/index.html

U.S. Office of the Assistant Secretary for Health. (2016). *National pain strategy: A comprehensive population health strategy for pain.* https://www.iprcc.nih.gov/sites/default/files/HHSNational_Pain_Strategy_508C.pdf

U.S. Office of the Surgeon General. (2016). *Facing addiction in America: The Surgeon General's report on alcohol, drugs, and health.* U.S. Department of Health and Human Services. https://www.ncbi.nlm.nih.gov/pubmed/28252892

U.S. Office of the Surgeon General. (2018). *Facing addiction in America: The Surgeon General's spotlight on opioids.* U.S. Department of Health and Human Services. https://addiction.surgeongeneral.gov/sites/default/files/OC_SpotlightOnOpioids.pdf

U.S. Department of Veterans Affairs and Department of Defense. (2017). *VA/DoD clinical practice guideline for opioid therapy for chronic pain* (Version 3.0).

U.S. Department of Veterans Affairs and Department of Defense. (2015). *VA/DoD clinical practice guideline for the management of substance use disorders.* https://www.healthquality.va.gov/guidelines/MH/sud/VADoDSUDCPGRevised22216.pdf

van Rijswijk, S. M., van Beek, M. H. C. T., Schoof, G. M., Schene, A. H., Steegers, M., & Schellekens, A. F. (2019). Iatrogenic opioid use disorder, chronic pain and psychiatric comorbidity: A systematic review. *General Hospital Psychiatry, 59*, 37–50. https://doi.org/10.1016/j.genhosppsych.2019.04.008

Veehof, M. M., Oskam, M.-J., Schreurs, K. M. G., & Bohlmeijer, E. T. (2011). Acceptance-based interventions for the treatment of chronic pain: A systematic review and meta-analysis. *Pain, 152*(3), 533–542. https://doi.org/10.1016/j.pain.2010.11.002

Vlaeyen, J. W., & Linton, S. J. (2000). Fear-avoidance and its consequences in chronic musculoskeletal pain: A state of the art. *Pain, 85*(3), 317–332. https://doi.org/10.1016/S0304-3959(99)00242-0

Von Korff, M., Kolodny, A., Deyo, R. A., & Chou, R. (2011). Long-term opioid therapy reconsidered. *Annals of Internal Medicine, 155*(5), 325–328. https://doi.org/10.7326/0003-4819-155-5-201109060-00011

Vowles, K. E., & McCracken, L. M. (2008). Acceptance and values-based action in chronic pain: A study of treatment effectiveness and process. *Journal of Consulting and Clinical Psychology, 76*(3), 397–407. https://doi.org/10.1037/0022-006X.76.3.397

Vowles, K. E., Witkiewitz, K., Cusack, K. J., Gilliam, W. P., Cardon, K. E., Bowen, S., Edwards, K. A., McEntee, M. L., & Bailey, R. W. (2019). Integrated behavioral treatment for Veterans with co-morbid chronic pain and hazardous opioid use: A randomized controlled pilot trial. *The Journal of Pain.* https://doi.org/10.1016/j.jpain.2019.11.007

Wager, T. D., Rilling, J. K., Smith, E. E., Sokolik, A., Casey, K. L., Davidson, R. J., Kosslyn, S. M., Rose, R. M., & Cohen, J. D. (2004). Placebo-induced changes in FMRI in the anticipation and experience of pain. *Science, 303*(5661), 1162–1167. https://doi.org/10.1126/science.1093065

Wampold, B. E. (2015). How important are the common factors in psychotherapy? An update. *World Psychiatry, 14*(3), 270–277. https://doi.org/10.1002/wps.20238

Wasan, A. D., Butler, S. F., Budman, S. H., Benoit, C., Fernandez, K., & Jamison, R. N. (2007). Psychiatric history and psychologic adjustment as risk factors for aberrant drug-related behavior among patients with chronic pain. *The Clinical Journal of Pain, 23*(4), 307–315. https://doi.org/10.1097/AJP.0b013e3180330dc5

Wasan, A. D., Michna, E., Edwards, R. R., Katz, J. N., Nedeljkovic, S. S., Dolman, A. J., Janfaza, D., Isaac, Z., & Jamison, R. N. (2015). Psychiatric comorbidity is associated prospectively with diminished opioid analgesia and increased opioid misuse in patients with chronic low back pain. *Anesthesiology, 123*(4), 861–872. https://doi.org/10.1097/ALN.0000000000000768

Washington Administrative Code 246-919-875 (2019). https://app.leg.wa.gov/wac/default.aspx?cite=246-919-870

Wertli, M. M., Eugster, R., Held, U., Steurer, J., Kofmehl, R., & Weiser, S. (2014). Catastrophizing—A prognostic factor for outcome in patients with low back pain: A systematic review. *The Spine Journal, 14*(11), 2639–2657. https://doi.org/10.1016/j.spinee.2014.03.003

Wertli, M. M., Rasmussen-Barr, E., Held, U., Weiser, S., Bachmann, L. M., & Brunner, F. (2014). Fear-avoidance beliefs—A moderator of treatment efficacy in patients with low back pain: A systematic review. *The Spine Journal, 14*(11), 2658–2678. https://doi.org/10.1016/j.spinee.2014.02.033

Williams, A. C. de C., Eccleston, C., & Morley, S. (2012). Psychological therapies for the management of chronic pain (excluding headache) in adults. *Cochrane Database of Systematic Reviews.* https://doi.org/10.1002/14651858.CD007407.pub3

Wilson, K. G., & Murrell, A. R. (2004). Values work in acceptance and commitment therapy. In S. C. Hayes, V. M. Follette, & M. Linehan (Eds.), *Mindfulness and acceptance: Expanding the cognitive-behavioral tradition* (pp. 120–151). Guilford Press.

Wollaars, M. M., Post, M. W. M., van Asbeck, F. W. A., & Brand, N. (2007). Spinal cord injury pain: The influence of psychologic factors and impact on quality of life. *The Clinical Journal of Pain, 23*(5), 383–391. https://doi.org/10.1097/AJP.0b013e31804463e5

Woolf, C. J. (2011). Central sensitization: Implications for the diagnosis and treatment of pain. *Pain, 152*(Suppl. 3), S2–S15. https://doi.org/10.1016/j.pain.2010.09.030

Woolf, S. H., & Schoomaker, H. (2019). Life expectancy and mortality rates in the United States, 1959–2017. *JAMA, 322*(20), 1996–2016. https://doi.org/10.1001/jama.2019.16932

World Health Organization (Ed.). (2009). *Clinical guidelines for withdrawal management and treatment of drug dependence in closed settings.* World Health Organization, Western Pacific Region.

Wu, T., Gao, X., Chen, M., van Dam, R. M., & the World Health Organization. (2009). Long-term effectiveness of diet-plus-exercise interventions vs. diet-only interventions for weight loss: A meta-analysis. *Obesity Reviews, 10*(3), 313–323. https://doi.org/10.1111/j.1467-789X.2008.00547.x

Yucha, C., & Montgomery, D. (2008). *Evidence-based practice in biofeedback and neurofeedback.* Association for Applied Psychophysiology and Biofeedback.

Zeidan, F., Grant, J. A., Brown, C. A., McHaffie, J. G., & Coghill, R. C. (2012). Mindfulness meditation-related pain relief: Evidence for unique brain mechanisms in the regulation of pain. *Neuroscience Letters, 520*(2), 165–173.

Zgierska, A. E., Burzinski, C. A., Cox, J., Kloke, J., Stegner, A., Cook, D. B., Singles, J., Mirgain, S., Coe, C. L., & Bačkonja, M. (2016). Mindfulness meditation and cognitive behavioral therapy intervention reduces pain severity and sensitivity in opioid-treated chronic low back pain: Pilot findings from a randomized controlled trial. *Pain Medicine, 17*(10), 1865–1881. https://doi.org/10.1093/pm/pnw006

Index

V

Veterans Health Administration, 137
Virtual reality, 90
Visualizations, 107
Von Korff, M., 18

W

Wall, P. D., 14–15, 17
Warmth of practitioner, 41
Wasan, A. D., 34

Washington State, xii
Water, pain flare-ups and, 121
Wellness-focused coping, 153–155
West Haven–Yale Multidimensional Pain
    Inventory, 93
Whole-person planning, 89–90
Withdrawal, 19, 23, 133–135

Z

Zgierska, A. E., 26

About the Authors

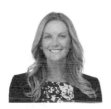

Jennifer L. Murphy, PhD, is a recognized authority and international speaker on optimizing behavioral treatments for chronic pain. She is the lead manual author, master trainer, and subject-matter expert for the Department of Veterans Affairs Cognitive Behavioral Therapy for Chronic Pain, and she is an associate professor at the University of South Florida's Morsani College of Medicine. In her long-term role as clinical director of Tampa VA's inpatient Chronic Pain Rehabilitation Program, Dr. Murphy provided clinical oversight for participants during opioid tapering. As a VA leader and active member of the American Academy of Pain Medicine, she has assisted in efforts to expand inclusion of behavioral health providers in pain care teams. Dr. Murphy is coinvestigator on numerous funded research trials, serves on the editorial board of *Pain Medicine*, and frequently authors peer-reviewed publications. Her knowledge and insights regarding nonpharmacological options to assist individuals with chronic pain have been used to positively impact research, education, and clinical care for individuals and systems in the public and private sectors. Visit her website (https://jennifermurphyphd.com/).

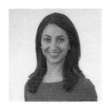

Samantha Rafie, PhD, is on the faculty at University of California San Diego Health, Department of Psychiatry and San Diego VA Healthcare System. Nationally, she is one of a small number of psychologists who are fellowship trained in chronic pain management, and she served veterans of the United States Armed Forces at the Tampa VA Chronic Pain Rehabilitation Program, the first in the country's VA health care system. Dr. Rafie serves as a consultant to functional restoration programs across California, providing specialized pain care to injured workers. Her clinical expertise extends from primary care pain management through tertiary-level pain rehabilitation programs, including opioid tapering, medication-assisted treatment, and detoxification. Dr. Rafie has authored numerous peer-reviewed publications and has trained interdisciplinary teams and future health care professionals in providing psychologically-informed pain care. Former chair of the ethics special interest group of the American Pain Society and founding member of the Alliance to Advance Comprehensive Integrative Pain Management's pain policy congress, Dr. Rafie strives to close existing gaps in pain treatment to improve care for those living with chronic pain. Visit her websites (https://www.samantharafiephd.com/ & https://mindoverpain.org) and follow @chronicpain_doc on Twitter.